MW01533651

HERPES CONTROLLED

~

≈

HERPES
CONTROLLED

New Drugs
New Strategies
New Solutions

≈

by
L. GRAY DAVIS, PhD,
CHARLES EBEL
JERRY STERN, MD

edited by
MICHAEL V. REITANO, MD,
LAWRENCE COREY, MD

Sexual Health Communications, Inc. ★ *Atlanta*

Manufactured in the U.S.A.
First edition, first printing

Library of Congress Catalog Card Number: 98-87166

ISBN 0-9666416-0-4

10 9 8 7 6 5 4 3 2 1

CONTENTS

Acknowledgments viii

Introduction 1

PART ONE

Cynthia's Story: Part One 9

chapter one
HERPES SIMPLEX VIRUSES IN PERSPECTIVE 19

1.1 Viruses: The Ultimate Parasites 19

1.2 Meet the Family 21

1.3 Human Herpesviruses 22

1.4 HSV-1 and HSV-2: Cut from the Same Cloth? 24

1.5 How HSV Infection Is Transmitted 25

    1.51 HSV-1 Transmission 26

    1.52 HSV-2 Transmission 27

1.6 How HSV Infection Is Established 28

    1.61 Inoculation, Replication, and Lesion Formation 28

    1.62 Latency, Reactivation, and Recurrence 30

1.7 The Antigenic Connection Between HSV-1 and HSV-2 31

1.8 The Three Forms of HSV Infection 35

1.9 Nongenital HSV Infections 36

PART TWO

Cynthia's Story: Part Two 39

chapter two
GENITAL HERPES: FACTS AND FIGURES 47

2.1 The Ongoing Epidemic: A Brief History 47

2.2 Epidemiology 49

2.21 HSV-1 or HSV-2? 50

2.22 Incidence and Prevalence of Genital Herpes 50

2.3 Transmission 52

2.4 Risk Factors 53

2.5 Symptoms 55

2.51 Symptomatic Primary Genital Herpes 57

2.52 Symptomatic Nonprimary Genital Herpes 60

2.53 Symptomatic Recurrent Genital Herpes 61

2.54 Prodromal Symptoms 62

2.6 Patterns of Recurrence 64

2.7 Diagnosis: What to Expect, What to Demand 65

2.71 A Complete History 65

2.72 Physical Examination 66

2.73 Testing for HSV 66

2.74 The Importance of Testing for Other STDs 69

2.8 Complications 69

2.9 Neonatal Herpes (HSV Infection in the Newborn) 71

2.91 Incidence and Acquisition 71

PART THREE

Cynthia's Story: Part Three 77

chapter three
GENITAL HERPES: TREATMENT, MANAGEMENT, AND
PREVENTION 85

3.1 How Did You Feel When You First Got the News? 85

3.2 Antiviral Therapy: What It Can and Can't Do 87

3.3 Treating the First Symptomatic Episode 88

3.4 Managing Recurrent Infection 91

*3.41 Episodic Antiviral Therapy for Recurrent
Genital Herpes 93*

*3.42 Suppressive Antiviral Therapy for Recurrent
Genital Herpes 95*

    3.43 Alternating Use of Episodic and Suppressive
           Antiviral Therapy 98

3.5 Prevention 100

    3.51 Single, Sexually Active, No Monogamous
           Relationship, and No History of Genital Herpes 100

    3.52 Single, Sexually Active, No Monogamous
           Relationship, and Diagnosed with Genital Herpes 102

    3.53 Monogamous Relationship, One Partner Has
           Genital Herpes 103

    3.54 Pregnant, No History of Genital Herpes 105

    3.55 Pregnant, Diagnosed with Genital Herpes 106

3.6 The Drug Approval Process and Alternative
    Medicines 106

    3.61 A Note on Lysine 109

3.7 Genital Herpes in the New Millennium 110

PART FOUR

Cynthia's Story: Epilogue 115

    chapter four
    GENITAL HERPES: QUESTIONS AND ANSWERS 121

    chapter five
    ADDITIONAL RESOURCES 137

Appendix A: Nongenital HSV Infections 147

Appendix B: Type-Specific Serologic Tests 153

Bibliography 157

Index 159

ACKNOWLEDGMENTS

The authors wish to thank the many people who have worked to improve public awareness of herpes or make better services available. A special thanks is owed to Simone Reitano, who conceived of and launched the New York–based Herpes Advice Center in 1984. Under her direction and inspired by her dedication to the concept of patient empowerment (long before it was fashionable), the Advice Center became nationally recognized as a center of excellence, paving the way for *Sexual Health* magazine and the Sexual Health Home Library.

This book also reflects the input of several talented writers, copy editors and proofreaders, chief among them Nicholas Puryear, whose insights and editorial skills were invaluable. Erin Willder coordinated all aspects of prepress work. Tom Orvald and Lisa Hyatt Smith provided administrative help during the formative stages of the project.

Medical illustrations were provided by Mike Dulude, with cover design by Colleen Carrigan and cover art by Andrea Cobb.

INTRODUCTION

~

Several years ago, a troupe of radio comedians called "Firesign Theater" released an album entitled *Everything You Know Is Wrong*. That would make a great title for a book about genital herpes. Most of what the average person in this country "knows" about genital herpes is from highly sensational press coverage in the late 1970s and early 1980s—the most famous example being *Time* magazine's 1982 cover story declaring herpes to be "The New Scarlet Letter." Such stories wrongly characterized genital herpes as a rare, severe disease and unfairly stigmatized the people who had it as sexual libertines. Back then, we doctors didn't know much about herpes either, but our knowledge has improved considerably over the past two decades. Consider, for example, the following points:

We used to think genital herpes was fairly uncommon, affecting no more than 1 in every 25 people in the United States. ⇨ **We now know** genital herpes is quite common, affecting roughly 1 in 4 persons 12 years of age or older in the United States— *about 45,000,000 people!*

We used to think genital herpes always produces extremely painful sores and other obvious symptoms. ⇨ **We now know** the vast majority of cases produce few symptoms or no symptoms whatsoever. In fact, in one study more than 90% of those who have genital herpes didn't even know they had it!

We used to think you could only get herpes by having sex with someone who had genital lesions at the time (rash, sores, blisters). ⇨ **We now know** 70% of people who get herpes get it from someone who has no lesions or other symptoms at the time.

We used to think because genital herpes is lifelong with unpredictable recurrences, you had to just "live with it" and suffer the consequences. ⇨ **We now know** with intelligent counseling, solid information, and strategic use of antiviral drugs, herpes can usually be controlled, and people with herpes can lead normal, happy lives.

TAKING CONTROL

As our knowledge of genital herpes has improved, our ideas about how it should be managed have changed. Today, we emphasize the patient's role: *It's your life. It's your infection. Who better than you to decide how it's going to be managed?* A doctor can educate you about the diagnosis, advise you on different strategies for herpes management, and prescribe the right treatment, but you will be the best judge of whether to use antiviral therapy and how and when to use it, once you understand the options.

Taking control of genital herpes also means taking control of your feelings about the disease. The potential psychosocial consequences of genital herpes — anger, fear, guilt, shame, depression, withdrawal, and social isolation — are perhaps less of a problem today than they were in the years before effective antiviral therapy. Nonetheless, many people are initially devastated to hear they have genital herpes, largely because of the associated stigma. Twenty years into the current epidemic, people with genital herpes are still the butt of jokes on television and in the movies. Granted, it's not the sort of intimate detail most people would want to reveal casually, but having genital herpes is nothing to be ashamed of either. It can happen to anyone, and it only takes one sexual encounter for a person to become infected.

Yes, genital herpes is a sexually transmitted disease. Yes, it can recur. But as we've said before and will say again and again: *Genital herpes can be controlled, and people with genital herpes can lead a normal, happy life.* No great sacrifices are required. There are certain precautions you can take to reduce the risk of transmission, but there's no reason why you can't have a fulfilling sex life, find love, marry, and raise a family, if that's your dream.

Some people with herpes feel they harbor a dark, dirty secret, and it gnaws away at their psyche. On this issue, the best counsel is to sharpen your appreciation of the difference between secrecy and privacy. You are certainly entitled to your privacy about herpes, but many find it's good to have at least one person to talk to — perhaps a close friend or a family member. Some find it helpful to attend meetings of a local herpes support group; there may be one organized in your area. These are personal decisions.

Telling your sexual partner about herpes is another matter. It can be complicated and awkward, but it is necessary and can even be helpful to a relationship. People with herpes who don't tell their partners often experience anxiety during what would otherwise be the pleasant, romantic, "getting-to-know-you" phase leading up to a sexual relationship. Fear of transmitting herpes can make sex itself feel like a deception. Every itch or odd sensation is magnified by the fear that it's the first manifestation of an outbreak. And what if an attack appears one or two days after a sexual encounter? Were you infectious at the time? Have you infected your partner?

The benefits of telling your partner are multiple. Once revealed, the risk of transmission becomes a shared responsibility. Openness dramatically reduces anxiety about transmission. It can also lead to an honest and clear discussion about STDs other than herpes. Remember there is at least a one-in-five chance your partner already has herpes. If so, there is a better than 90 percent chance he or she doesn't even know it. A special type-specific blood test could answer this question, and we'll explain what that is and how to obtain one later in the book. Herpes isn't "ping-ponged" back and forth between partners, so finding out whether your partner has a "silent" herpes infection would eliminate your anxiety over transmission.

HOW TO USE THIS BOOK

You'll find more information here than is needed to avoid, understand, or control a genital herpes infection. But one of our goals is to dispel some of the myth and stigma associated with herpes, and the best antidote for that sort of misinformation is a healthy dose of fact. If you are a person with herpes and you intend to have a normal, active sex life, you will need to share some of these facts with prospective partners.

The book is organized primarily as a handbook. The sections and subsections within each chapter are numbered for quick access and easy reference. For example: Chapter 2.0, "Genital Herpes: Facts and Figures," contains section 2.5, "Symptoms," which contains subsection 2.51, "Symptomatic Primary Genital Herpes."

Chapter 1 discusses the two viruses that can cause genital herpes (HSV-1 and HSV-2) in the larger context of the herpesvirus family and viruses in general. It outlines the differences and, most important, the similarities between HSV-1 and HSV-2. It explains how both viruses are spread and profiles the principal nongenital infections they can cause.

Chapter 2 focuses exclusively on genital herpes: its distribution in the population, risk factors for acquisition, symptoms, patterns of recurrence, diagnosis, complications, and risks to pregnant women and their newborn babies.

Chapter 3 opens with a discussion of the psychosocial effects of diagnosis and recurrent disease and goes on to explain the treatment of initial episodes of infection and strategies for managing recurrent infection, including how to help prevent transmission to partners. New directions in drug and vaccine research are also reviewed.

Chapter 4 presents and answers some of the most frequently asked questions about genital herpes and could be used as a self-test to measure your knowledge of genital herpes before and after reading the book.

Chapter 5 lists a number of resources for additional information and support.

SAY HELLO TO CYNTHIA

Interspersed between chapters, you'll find a running narrative — the story of Cynthia, a young professional woman, whose fictional experience of genital herpes is based on the actual experience of numerous real-life patients we have listened to, treated, and counseled over the years. Cynthia's story is chiefly meant to show the profound effect a surprise diagnosis of genital herpes can have on a person and his or her relationships. It is also intended to illuminate the very important concept of asymptomatic viral shedding, the principal mechanism by which the modern epidemic of genital herpes has been, and continues to be, sustained. But it is also a human story of how one person comes to grips with a herpes diagnosis and uses accurate information to manage her disease and get on with her life.

A NOTE ON REFERENCES

Much of the factual information in this book was culled from selected chapters in four contemporary texts:

- Corey L. "Herpes Simplex Virus." In: Fauci AS, Braunwald E, Isselbacher KJ, eds. *Harrison's Principles of Internal Medicine.* 14th ed. New York, NY: McGraw-Hill, Inc; 1997.
- Corey L. "Genital Herpes." In: Holmes KH, Mårdh P-A, Stamm WE, Sparling PF, eds. *Sexually Transmitted Diseases.* 3rd ed. New York, NY: McGraw-Hill, Inc; 1998.
- Roizman B. "The Family Herpesviridae" and Whitley RJ, Gnann JW. "The Epidemiology and Clinical Manifestations of Herpes Simplex Virus Infections." In: Roizman B, Whitley RJ, Lopez C, eds. *The Human Herpesviruses.* New York, NY: Raven Press; 1993.

- Oxman MN. "Genital Herpes" and "Herpes Simplex Viruses and Human Herpesvirus 6." In: Gorbach SL, Bartlett JG, Blacklow NR, eds. *Infectious Diseases.* Philadelphia, PA: W. B. Saunders Company; 1992.

These chapters draw upon many hundreds of clinical studies and scientific papers, and a listing of each source document cited is not feasible. However, a debt of medical scholarship to the authors and editors of each is gratefully acknowledged. Throughout this book, reference to specific studies is made with the lead author's name and the date of publication in parentheses, e.g. (Corey 1994), and the complete bibliography, for all chapters, begins on page 157.

If you have genital herpes, our greatest hope is that this book will prove useful in your efforts to understand and manage your disease and to avoid transmitting it to your sexual partners. It's crucial that you not define yourself in terms of your disease. Yes, you have herpes, but you are not a "herpetic." Herpes is *not* who you are.

In our experience of treating many thousands of patients, we've found that the vast majority are well and happy. Among those who are not, the reason seldom has anything to do with herpes.

part
ONE

Cynthia's Story:

*One Woman's Experience
with Genital Herpes*

❧

Cynthia was an attractive 29-year-old graphic designer, working for a busy advertising agency in midtown Manhattan. She'd come to New York from Minnesota, fresh out of college, in June of 1989. Her early years in the city were devoted to building a career, which left only minimal time for a social life. She dated intermittently and had two or three sexual relationships, but none that lasted more than six months. For the past four years, however, she'd been in a mutually monogamous relationship with Brian, a 35-year-old litigator at one of the city's older and more prestigious law firms.

She met Brian in May of 1992, at an awards dinner for a celebrity tennis tournament. His firm was one of the corporate sponsors, and her agency had volunteered to handle the advertising and promotion. They started dating, and right away, everything just seemed to click. They were "outdoorsy" and athletic; they shared similar tastes in food, music, and movies; and they both wanted children. Brian was a native New Yorker, quite sophisticated in Cynthia's eyes, but he was also attentive and romantic and had a great sense of humor. The sexual aspects of their relationship were, as far as Cynthia was concerned, perfect.

Happy together, careers firmly on track, they felt the time was right for marriage and a family, so at the end of the summer, they announced their engagement and set a tentative date for the following June.

Cynthia had always paid close attention to her health and fitness. She watched her diet and worked out regularly. Once a year, she had a routine physical examination and a Pap smear. In her entire life, she had slept with only six different men, including Brian. Her sexual health was generally excellent; her Pap smears had always been negative; and she'd never had any serious gynecological problems. In college, she'd been plagued by recurrent yeast infection, but since moving to New York, that seemed to have more or less resolved. The occasional flare-up was easily controlled with an over-the-counter medication, miconazole.

The Thursday evening after Labor Day, around ten o'clock, Cynthia was lying alone in bed watching television when she noticed a vague burning and itching sensation in her vaginal area. Her first thought was that she was getting another yeast infection. Over the long holiday weekend, she and Brian had been especially amorous in anticipation of his leaving town for two weeks to argue a case in San Diego. It was not unusual for her to develop a yeast infection after a period of vigorous sexual activity. Within an hour, the vague discomfort progressed to intense vaginal pain. Cynthia got up, went into the bathroom, and rummaged through a drawer until she found the miconazole. She always kept a tube handy for just such an emergency.

Cynthia didn't sleep well. She was in constant pain and had to get up over and over to urinate. As the night wore on, the act of urination itself became increasing painful. By morning she was determined to see her gynecologist. She phoned Dr. Charles's office and related her symptoms to one of the nurses. The nurse agreed that Cynthia's pain was excessive for a yeast infection and suggested she come in for a quick examination on her way to work. They would squeeze her in somehow.

When she arrived, the reception area was packed with other women, many of them pregnant, but Cynthia didn't have to wait. A nurse escorted her to an examining room and asked her to change into a gown and have a seat on the table. Then she slipped a thermometer into Cynthia's mouth. "I'll be right back," she said, and a few minutes later, she returned with the doctor.

Dr. Charles removed the thermometer from Cynthia's mouth, studied it briefly, and handed it to the nurse. Then he picked up Cynthia's file from the countertop. "You've got a bit of a fever," he said casually, leafing through her file. "What seems to be wrong?"

"I feel like hell," Cynthia said. "I've been up all night." And she told him about the vaginal pain, the urinary problems, and the aching in her groin that had begun earlier that morning. "At first I thought it was just another yeast infection, but now I don't know. It hurts so bad." Dr. Charles nodded. He made a note in her file and set it back down on the countertop. Then he donned a pair of latex gloves and took up his usual position on a small wheeled stool at the foot of the table.

The examination took longer than usual, and when Cynthia realized this, her anxiety started to build. Something was wrong, she just knew it. When Dr. Charles asked the nurse for a large magnifying glass, Cynthia propped herself up on her elbows, trying to see what was happening. And when he asked for sterile swabs and "culture material," she couldn't help but see the look of concern on the nurse's face. "This is going to hurt," Dr. Charles said, apologetically, "but it'll be over in a second." Cynthia winced as he swabbed first her left and then her right labia. "I'm sorry," he said, handing the swabs back to the nurse, "That's all. All done." He removed his latex examination gloves and dropped them in a red trash container marked *Infectious/Hazardous Waste*. Cynthia had never noticed the container before. Now she couldn't take her eyes from it.

She sat up on the table and smoothed the paper gown out across her thighs. Dr. Charles swiveled around to face her and, after a moment's hesitation, said "I'm afraid I have some rather alarming news for you, but I don't want you to panic, okay?" She nodded half-heartedly.

"I believe you have genital herpes." Dr. Charles said, gently. He paused, trying to gauge Cynthia's reaction, but she just stared blankly at the floor. "In fact, I'm sure of it," he continued in a slightly apologetic tone. "I've seen a lot of herpes, and this is a classic case. We'll send your culture to a lab for confirmation, but regardless of the results, that's my diagnosis. It's a pretty severe case, actually, which makes me think it's probably a primary first episode. . . ."

He went on to explain what "primary first episode" meant, but Cynthia didn't hear anything he said after "herpes." *That* was not a word she had ever expected to hear from her doctor.

Herpes! Her mind was racing, and she felt a cold rush of adrenaline in her stomach and legs — the sudden onset of panic and dread. *Herpes? How could I have herpes?* She was trying to recall what she had read or heard about herpes and whether she'd ever known anyone who'd had it. All she could remember for sure was it was some kind of venereal disease, like gonorrhea or syphilis. And for some reason, the phrase "occupational hazard of prostitutes" kept running through her head.

Dr. Charles swiveled back around to the countertop, wrote something on a small pad of paper, and tore the top sheet away. "Here's a prescription," he said. "This will help with the pain, and it will help clear up the current infection. I want you to take one of these capsules five times a day for the next ten days — one at eight in the morning, one at noon, one at four, one at eight in the evening, and one at midnight or at bedtime. They're very safe, and after your follow-up visit we'll talk about strategies for managing recurrence."

"Recurrence?" Cynthia whispered in anguished disbelief.

Dr. Charles nodded. "But recurrent infections usually aren't so painful and usually don't last as long as primary episodes. Make an appointment for a follow-up visit ten days from now," he continued. "The culture results will be back by then, and we'll talk." He glanced at his watch. "There are things you need to know about pregnancy and cancer risk that we don't have time to discuss now. I'm *really* sorry." On his way to the door, he touched Cynthia's hand and said, reassuringly, "I know this may seem like the end of the world, but it isn't. It's not as bad as you think, honest. I'll see you in ten days, okay?" He waited for her to make eye contact, then added, sympathetically, "Please, do not let this get you into a panic. It's not that big a deal, I promise. I'll see you in ten days, okay? Are you going to be okay?" Cynthia nodded. Dr. Charles asked the nurse to take a blood sample and left the room.

Cynthia didn't even realize she was crying until the nurse handed her a tissue. "It's a shock, isn't it?" the nurse said. "Are you up for this?" She was holding a rubber tourniquet and a blood-sample tube.

"What's that for?" Cynthia asked, slightly alarmed.

"I need to take a blood sample," the nurse replied. "But we can wait a minute or two." Cynthia wiped the tears from her cheeks and blew her nose. The shock of the diagnosis had left her feeling lightheaded and a little nauseated. It must have shown. "Why don't you take a couple of minutes to pull yourself together," the nurse said, patting her on the shoulder. "I'll go schedule your follow-up. Is Monday after next, first thing in the morning, okay?" Cynthia just nodded. "We also have some literature that will help explain more." The nurse retrieved some pamphlets from a drawer and handed them to Cynthia.

Sitting there alone, in that flimsy paper gown, with a damp tissue in one hand and a fistful of pamphlets in the other, Cynthia began to feel that she too was somehow tainted and disposable — dirty and used. *Infectious/Hazardous Waste* she read again, staring at the red trash container. She desperately wanted more time with Dr. Charles, but she also knew she'd been squeezed in this morning at the last possible minute. She sincerely appreciated the special consideration, but she needed more time. Her mind was starting to fill up with questions. *How could I have herpes? What have I done to deserve this? What did he mean about cancer and pregnancy? When is this going to come back?* Then she thought of Brian. *Oh my God, could I have given this to Brian?* And a moment later, a darker thought came to her, *Could Brian have given it to me? Has he been unfaithful?*

The nurse returned about five minutes later. When she finished taking the blood sample, she offered Cynthia a few more encouraging words and said they would see her in a couple of weeks. Cynthia dressed hurriedly, paid her bill, and left.

～

By the time she reached the street, Cynthia had made up her mind not to go in to work. She was exhausted from the sleepless night before, and totally preoccupied with the news of her diagnosis. There was no way she could hide her distress from her co-workers, and she was not about to tell anyone at work she had herpes. Over the years she'd heard plenty of jokes and snide comments about herpes and little in the way of compassion for those who had it. She wanted someone to talk to, but couldn't think who to call. Her family was out of the question; that would just be too embarrassing. Besides, she was in no mood for the predictable lecture about New York City and the veritable Babylon it represented to her overprotective parents. She headed for the subway, but the vaginal pain was excruciating. Walking just made it worse, so she hailed a cab. But she had the driver stop four blocks from the apartment so she could fill the prescription at a pharmacy where neither she nor Brian normally shopped.

When she got back to the apartment, she phoned the agency and told her supervisor she had a stomach virus and could not come in today, possibly not Monday either. He made a joke about long weekends and sick leave, but told her to take care of herself and not to worry.

She took one of the capsules Dr. Charles had prescribed. Then she undressed, pulled on a pair of sweat pants and one of Brian's old T-shirts, and crawled into bed. Her mind was still racing. She couldn't shake the thought that Brian might have been unfaithful. How else could she have gotten this? She hadn't slept with anyone else since they'd met. She and Brian no longer used condoms, having both tested negative for HIV when they decided to move in together, but every other man she'd slept with had worn a condom, *with nonoxynol;* she had always insisted on it. No, there had to be a better explanation. Brian would never cheat on her. She felt a twinge of guilt for even harboring the thought.

The next week passed quickly for Cynthia, and by Friday, she was feeling much better, physically. The vaginal pain and urinary problems were gone. The depression and listlessness that had driven her to bed the previous weekend had lifted, but emotionally, she was still fragile. Brian had called each night before she went to bed, but she never mentioned her visit to Dr. Charles.

Just before lunch, the nurse from Dr. Charles's office phoned to say all of Cynthia's test results had come back negative. The viral culture was negative, but the doctor was fairly certain it was a "false negative." The term meant nothing to Cynthia, but she understood that her diagnosis had not changed. She still had herpes.

The nurse then asked Cynthia a few questions about her infection: Had the lesions started to heal? And how was she feeling otherwise? Cynthia told her the pain and the urinary problems were gone, as well as the fever and headaches, and that she was getting to sleep and staying asleep without difficulty. Overall, she felt much better.

"That's good. That's real good," the nurse said. "Another thing," she continued. "Dr. Charles can't see you on Monday. He had to put one of his obstetric patients in the hospital today. It was an emergency."

Cynthia's heart sank, but she said nothing.

"They're going to do a C-section, but not until Monday morning. There are some tests they have to run first. It's a complicated case. Anyway, he needs to leave Monday open. I've been here all afternoon rescheduling his appointments. But everything seems to be going okay with you. That's good. Can I reschedule you for Friday, October 4th?"

Cynthia couldn't believe it. "That's three weeks from now!" she protested.

"I know," the nurse replied, sympathetically.

"Well, I need to talk to him before then. Can't you do any better than October? Please? Don't you have anything next week? Anything? I'll come whenever he can see me." Cynthia was trying to imagine how she could put off sex with Brian for three weeks. What could she tell him?

"Let's see," the nurse said slowly. "Let's take a look here." Cynthia heard the nurse tapping rhythmically on a computer keyboard. "I think we could squeeze you in for thirty minutes sometime near the end of the month. How does Friday, the 27th, at 8 a.m. look for you? That's the week after next."

"That's not soon enough," Cynthia pleaded. "And thirty minutes? That's not enough time, is it?" She was rapidly moving from frustration to anger, but if she lost her temper now, the floodgates would open, and she didn't want a tearful scene at work. Besides, it wasn't the nurse's fault, and there was no point arguing. "Is there any chance I could speak to Dr. Charles now?" she asked politely, resigning herself to this latest disappointment.

"No. I'm sorry. He's not here. He's been at the hospital since around ten this morning. Would you like to leave a message?"

"No," Cynthia said, "that's okay. Put me down for the 27th at eight."

As if losing her Monday appointment with Dr. Charles weren't enough, Brian called later that Friday afternoon to say he would be home the next day. The defendants in the suit he was preparing had decided to settle out of court.

"I miss you," he said, lovingly. "What's it been, almost two weeks? I haven't been able to stop thinking about our Labor Day weekend. I can't wait to see you."

Cynthia's resolve not to obsess, not to panic, was beginning to crumble. She had counted on being able to talk to Dr. Charles *before* Brian got back. Now what was she supposed to do? Sex any time soon was definitely out of the question. Sex was the last thing she wanted to think about. And she still didn't know how or what to tell Brian, *or ask him.*

∿

Brian returned on Saturday around 5:30 p.m. When he made sexual overtures later that evening, Cynthia sweetly but firmly declined. Out of desperation, she told him she was getting a yeast infection. She hated to lie, but what else could she do? She simply was not ready to tell him the truth. In this case, she could honestly say she didn't know the truth, at least not the whole truth. Better to wait until she had more information than to bring this up and find herself unable to answer the inevitable flurry of questions. She decided she would continue using the "yeast defense" for a few more days, at least until she figured out what to do next.

On Sunday, while reading the paper, she noticed an ad from the Midtown Women's Clinic—*DO YOU HAVE GENITAL HERPES?* She read it carefully. The Clinic was recruiting couples to participate in vaccine research. There was a number to call. Maybe this vaccine could help? If they were doing herpes research, she might at least be able to get some answers. So the first thing she did Monday morning was phone the Clinic and schedule an appointment. She mentioned her interest in the vaccine and was told she would need to talk to Dr. Foster. He could see her Wednesday morning. Cynthia said she had only recently been diagnosed with herpes and still had a lot of questions. "I'll put you down for an hour," the woman at the clinic said, "and if you need more time after that, we'll get you back in a few days. How's that?"

"That," Cynthia said smiling, "would be just great."

Finally. Some answers.

chapter one

HERPES SIMPLEX VIRUSES IN PERSPECTIVE

~

1.1 VIRUSES: THE ULTIMATE PARASITES

Viruses are important causes of illness in humans. AIDS, Ebola, mumps, polio, warts, herpes, rabies, measles, smallpox, influenza, yellow fever, and the common cold are all caused by different viruses.

Viruses present us with some of our toughest medical challenges. A handful of viral disease are largely controllable with vaccines, most notably influenza, polio, chickenpox, and smallpox. And a relatively small number can be either cured or managed with drug therapy. But the majority of viral infections, like the classic 24-hour stomach virus or the common cold, are untreatable and self-limiting. Your doctor tells you to get plenty of rest, drink plenty of fluids, and maybe take aspirin or acetaminophen for pain or to reduce the fever. But the infection must be allowed simply to burn itself out, which is another way of saying the body's immune system eventually triumphs.

Viruses can be regarded as parasites because they depend entirely on a host organism for their continued existence. And although we use the terms "alive" and "killed" to describe the ability of a quantity of virus to cause infection, viruses barely qualify as living organisms because they cannot perform any of the normal functions of life on their own. Outside of a cell, they simply exist, neither benign nor malignant.

They cannot reproduce, convert food into energy, or even make their own structural components.

The individual virus unit or particle, which we call a **virion,** consists mainly of a single molecule of nucleic acid ("the code of life"), either DNA or RNA, surrounded by protein. A virion has none of the characteristics that typify a plant or animal cell. It has no nucleus—the "command center" that regulates cellular activity. And it has no organelles—the cell's equivalent of internal organs, which carry out the tasks of respiration and elimination.

Viruses make their way in the world by invading healthy cells in a host organism and changing the cell's operating instructions—"rewriting the cellular software," so to speak. An infected cell is thus tricked into manufacturing DNA (or RNA) and proteins for the virus instead of the normal cellular products the cell needs for its own growth and division. New virions are assembled inside the infected cell using the cell's energy. Eventually, the infected cell bursts or disintegrates, releasing a large number of newly manufactured virions that take over other healthy cells, and the infectious process continues.

In some cases, the host dies as a result of the infection—sometimes quickly, as with Ebola; sometimes over a period of several years, as with AIDS. In other cases, drug therapy cures the infection, or the host's natural defenses rally to combat and eliminate the virus. In the case of herpesviruses, however, the normal course of infection is strikingly different: the signs and symptoms of infection may disappear, but *all herpesviruses are capable of establishing a **latent** infection—one that persists for the life of the natural host and may be reactivated later.*

If you think about it from the virus's perspective, the longer it stays in the host and avoids being destroyed by the host, the better its odds of being transmitted to someone else. If a virus overtakes its host too quickly, and the host succumbs before it can spread the virus to someone else, then the virus's "life" also ends. This is why we have yet to see rapid expansion of Ebola—those who are infected tend to die before they can travel a significant distance and pass the virus on to others.

1.2 MEET THE FAMILY

Almost all amphibian, reptilian, and mammalian species are infected with a herpesvirus. Each of these herpesviruses is adapted to its particular host. Birds, cats, cows, dogs, elephants, fish, frogs, hedgehogs, horses, lizards, mice, monkeys, pigs, rats, rabbits, reindeer, seals, sheep, snakes, squirrels, turtles, wallabies, woodchucks, and wildebeests — all have their own unique "brand" of herpes.

An interesting feature of all herpesviruses is that under the electron microscope they look quite similar. All share a common and elegantly simple architecture (see Figure 1.2).

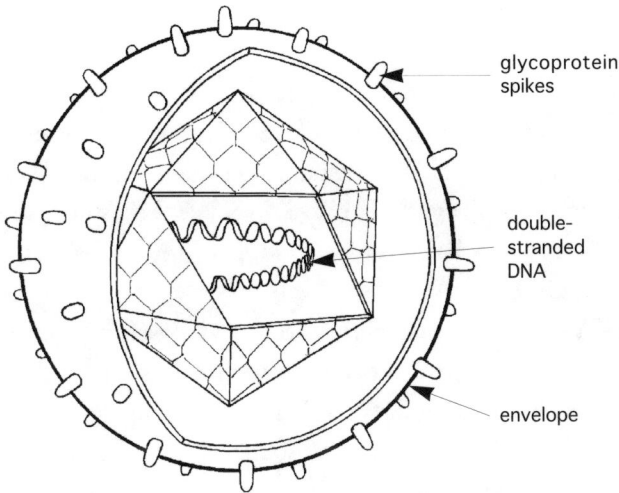

glycoprotein spikes

double-stranded DNA

envelope

FIGURE 1.2 **Herpesvirus virion** —The core contains a single molecule of viral DNA connected end-to-end in a wreath- or donut-like form and is protected by a protein **capsid** made up of 162 identical **capsomeres.** The uniformity of the capsomere streamlines the production of new virions. Geometrically speaking, the capsid is a regular icosadeltahedron, which means it has twenty equilateral triangular sides. Surrounding the capsid is another layer of viral protein called the **tegument.** The tegument is enclosed by the **envelope,** which the virion scavenges from the nuclear membrane of the infected host cell. Embedded in the envelope and radiating outwardly from its surface are hundreds of tiny **glycoprotein spikes.** The spikes enable the virion to attach itself to a host cell and penetrate the cell's protective outer membrane.

As mentioned before, all herpesviruses can become dormant or latent in the infected host and then be reactivated later. The site or cell type within the body where latency is established varies. Herpes simplex viruses (HSV-1 and HSV-2) establish latency in nerve cells, but Epstein-Barr virus, another human herpesvirus, establishes latency in a type of white blood cell, the B lymphocyte.

Knowing that herpes simplex viruses hide in nerve cells can help us understand why HSV infection is lifelong. The body does not use its considerable inflammatory capacity to rid itself of infection in the nervous system because once nerve tissue is destroyed, it cannot regenerate. Other tissues, such as skin, are replaced after injury, but a lost nerve cell is lost forever.

1.3 HUMAN HERPESVIRUSES

There are eight known human herpesviruses: herpes simplex virus-1 (HSV-1); herpes simplex virus-2 (HSV-2); varicella-zoster virus (VZV); Epstein-Barr virus (EBV); human cytomegalovirus (CMV); and human herpesviruses 6, 7, and 8 (HHV-6, HHV-7, HHV-8). Although some of the names may be new to you, some of the diseases associated with them should be familiar.

HSV-1 is the human herpesvirus most closely associated with infections of the mouth and throat, especially cold sores on the lips. **HSV-2** is the principal cause of genital herpes. Both viruses can also cause eye infection, central nervous system problems, and other kinds of skin infection. For the most part, HSV infection is a mild condition, but it can sometimes be life-threatening in newborns and in people whose immune systems are compromised. **Immunocompromise** is most commonly seen in patients with severe burns; in patients with HIV infection and AIDS; in patients undergoing chemotherapy for cancer; and in the recipients of transplanted body organs (when it is chemically induced to prevent rejection of the transplant).

Table 1.3 summarizes the human herpesviruses and their associated diseases.

Table 1.3   The Human Herpesviruses

	Mainly associated with	*Also associated with*
Herpes simplex virus-1 (HSV-1)	Cold sores on the lip; other infections of the mouth and throat	Eye infection; central nervous system infection (herpes simplex encephalitis); various infections in newborns and the immunocompromised (patients with burns, organ transplants, HIV, or AIDS); misc. skin infections, including infection of the finger
Herpes simplex virus-2 (HSV-2)	Genital herpes	Central nervous system infection (herpes simplex meningitis); various infections in newborns and immunocompromised patients; misc. skin infections
Varicella zoster virus (VZV)	Chickenpox and shingles	Infections in immunocompromised patients
Epstein-Barr virus (EBV)	Mononucleosis ("mono")	Several cancers of the lymphatic system; infections in immunocompromised patients
Cytomegalovirus (CMV)	Mononucleosis (but only about 8% of cases)	Various infections in newborns and immunocompromised patients, especially those with HIV/AIDS
Human herpesvirus 6 (HHV-6)	Roseola infantum (aka pseudorubella, exanthema subitum, or "sixth disease")	Infections in immunocompromised patients
Human herpesvirus 7 (HHV-7)	No known diseases	Unknown
Human herpesvirus 8 (HHV-8)	Kaposi's sarcoma (AIDS- and non–AIDS-related)	Rare disease of lymph cells

1.4 HSV-1 and HSV-2:
Cut from the Same Cloth?

It is often said that HSV-1 strikes above the waist, and HSV-2 strikes below the waist. While fundamentally true, this is an overstatement. HSV-1 and HSV-2 are closely related, and their roles as infectious agents overlap significantly: HSV-1, though mainly the cause of herpes infection in and about the mouth, has become a frequent cause of genital infection; HSV-2, though mainly the cause of genital herpes, can also cause oral infection.

How did this phenomenon of two viruses with separate but overlapping lifestyles evolve? There is evidence that HSV-1 and HSV-2 descended from a common ancestor some 8 to 10 million years ago. The ancient HSV progenitor is believed to have been similar to *Herpesvirus simiae,* a herpesvirus that infects several species of monkey. Nearly all susceptible monkeys in the wild are infected with *Herpesvirus simiae.* Direct and indirect oral-genital contact is a common feature of the sexual and grooming behaviors of monkeys, and *Herpesvirus simiae* depends equally on oral and genital routes for transmission.

Theoretically, as our early ancestors began to adopt an upright, two-legged stance and a face-to-face mating position, oral and genital areas were more effectively separated from each other. This led to a decrease in the frequency of oral-genital contact and thus created a kind of microbiological isolation to allow HSV-1 and HSV-2 to evolve at their "preferred" anatomic sites of infection. This process is believed to have been aided by another development in human evolution that is thought to have occurred around the same time: the extension of female sexual attractiveness across the entire menstrual cycle, as opposed to just those few days in the month when conception is most likely. This meant more frequent mating, and more frequent mating meant more opportunities for infection to spread — a condition necessary to maintain the evolving herpes simplex viruses in the population over time.

Further evidence that HSV-1 and HSV-2 are naturally adapted to their preferred sites of infection is seen in their patterns of recurrence. One of the signal features of HSV infection is that the latent virus can become reactivated periodically, causing a recurrence of disease. But genital herpes caused by HSV-1 is far less likely to recur than genital herpes caused by HSV-2, and oral infection caused by HSV-2 is much less likely to recur than oral infection caused by HSV-1. An infection that is less likely to recur is also less likely to be passed on to a new host. For millions of years, then, HSV-1 and HSV-2 have been able to maintain the essential separation of their preferred sites of infection, despite the fact that they are physically capable of causing infection at either site. Interestingly, in the decades following the sexual revolution, an increase in oral-genital sexual activity has led to an increase in the number of cases of genital herpes caused by HSV-1. We'll discuss that phenomenon later.

1.5 HOW HSV INFECTION IS TRANSMITTED

Some infectious diseases are transmitted through the air — a person sneezes, expelling aerosolized droplets of infected respiratory secretion; another person breathes in those droplets and becomes infected. Influenza viruses are spread in this fashion. Other infectious diseases are transmitted when a person comes in contact with contaminated environmental surfaces. Many bacterial infections are spread in this manner — salmonella, from chicken residue on a kitchen sink or countertop, for example. Still other infections are transmitted by animals — rats, mice, fleas, ticks, mosquitoes, etc. We associate malaria with mosquitoes and Lyme disease with ticks. The deadly Hanta virus has been traced to the droppings of deer mice, and the rabies virus is spread from the saliva of infected animals, usually as the result of a bite. None of these modes of transmission applies to HSV.

HSV infection, whether it is caused by HSV-1 or HSV-2, results (almost always) from direct skin-to-skin/body-to-body contact, when active virus from an infected person is brought into direct contact with the susceptible skin or other tissues of an uninfected person.

The susceptible tissue is often mucous membrane — the soft, moist lining inside the mouth, vagina, urethra, and rectum. The delicate tissues of the vulva, penis, and scrotum are also susceptible. Intact **epidermis,** like the skin on our hands, arms, legs, and torso, is more resistant to

HSV infection, but a minor cut or scrape or a skin condition like eczema can leave the skin vulnerable. Even a microscopic break in genital tissues resulting from sexual intercourse can provide an adequate portal for the entry of HSV.

Herpes infections are not airborne and are not spread by insects or animals. And although HSV has been shown in the laboratory to "survive" on environmental surfaces for several hours, acquisition by contact with inanimate objects — doorknobs, toilet seats, hot tubs, swimming pools, or contaminated towels — is extremely unlikely. There are no documented cases attributed to this mode of transmission. HSV quickly loses its ability to cause infection when exposed to the air, heat, solvents, detergents, extremes of pH, or protein-destroying enzymes.

1.51 HSV-1 Transmission

Because the associated infections occur primarily in and around the mouth, HSV-1 is usually transmitted in saliva. Any action or activity that allows the infected saliva of one person to come into contact with the susceptible tissues of another person presents an opportunity for infection. HSV-1 can be spread by kissing. Drinking from the same glass or bottle immediately after someone with an active infection (or someone who is shedding virus asymptomatically in his or her saliva) is another possible way to acquire HSV-1. If you've ever observed young children at play and seen how frequently they put their fingers in their mouths and touch the faces of other children, it shouldn't surprise you to learn that primary HSV-1 infection often occurs in childhood.

The likelihood of HSV-1 infection is inversely related to socioeconomic status, which is to say that crowded living conditions (especially in childhood) and poor hygiene favor the spread of HSV-1. Interestingly, childhood HSV-1 infection in the United States has been on the decline in recent decades. This decline is attributed in part to the increasing use of paper and plastic cups and the increasing use of electric dishwashers — both of which decrease the sharing of cups and glasses.

Genital herpes due to HSV-1 is frequently the result of oral-genital contact. However, it is possible to transfer HSV-1 from the mouth to the genitals by hand, such as when saliva is used as a sexual lubricant.

Genital-to-genital transmission is also possible, although the recurrence rate for genital herpes due to HSV-1 is relatively low, which means the opportunities for transmission are comparatively reduced.

In addition, there is a relatively uncommon form of nongenital HSV infection called **herpetic whitlow,** a painful infection of the fingertip. The usual portal of entry for the virus in cases of herpetic whitlow is thought to be a cut or fissure in the cuticle of the fingernail. Herpetic whitlow can be caused by HSV-1 or HSV-2 and has long been recognized as an occupational hazard of health care professionals, especially dentists and dental hygienists, whose hands are frequently in contact with the contaminated saliva of infected patients. In a small number of cases, those experiencing a primary genital herpes episode might also develop whitlow as a result of touching their own herpes lesions. (This phenomenon, called **autoinoculation,** is discussed in Appendix A.) It's important to note that autoinoculation is a concern only in a primary episode; antibodies and other immune responses develop within several months of the primary infection, making autoinoculation during recurrent episodes extremely unlikely. As a precaution, we counsel patients to avoid touching their lesions during a primary episode and to wash their hands if they do touch them.

1.52 HSV-2 Transmission

HSV-2 infections are predominantly genital infections, and the spread of HSV-2 is related mainly to sexual activity. Any sexual activity that brings susceptible tissue of an uninfected person into direct contact with the genitals, or the area surrounding the genitals, of an infected person presents an opportunity for the transmission of HSV-2. Contact can be genital-genital, oral-genital, genital-anal, or oral-anal.

Recalling our "skin-to-skin/body-to-body" rule for HSV transmission, you've probably already surmised that an oral HSV-2 infection can be acquired through oral sex, either cunnilingus or fellatio. Just as HSV-1 can be spread via the liquid medium of saliva, HSV-2 can be spread by vaginal secretions and semen. Oral HSV-2 infection could also be passed from person to person by the same means that oral HSV-1 is spread, in contaminated saliva, but this mode of transmission is probably relatively uncommon because the recurrence rate for oral HSV-2 infection is so low.

1.6 How HSV Infection Is Established

In about 80 percent of cases, initial infection with HSV produces no recognized symptoms, and latency is established without the infected person ever knowing he or she has acquired herpes. In other cases, signs and symptoms of varying intensity are present. The complete course of lesion formation is described below, but it bears repeating that most people infected with HSV have no lesions or only mild lesions that are easily mistaken for something harmless like heat rash, jock itch, a pimple, an ingrown hair, or a yeast infection.

1.61 Inoculation, Replication, and Lesion Formation

The first step in HSV infection is **inoculation,** when virus is deposited on a mucosal surface or gains access to the skin through a cut, burn, abrasion, or other disruption in the outermost layer of the skin. HSV replication begins near the site of inoculation in an internal layer of skin. Infected cells disintegrate, releasing more virus to attack neighboring cells. In general terms, HSV causes changes in the skin or mucous membranes, such as the vaginal lining. These changes, called **lesions** when they are visible, take many forms, as previously stated, ranging from simple redness to tiny pimple-like sores to blisters and open ulcers. The classic lesion is depicted in Figure 1.61.

When lesions form on mucosal surfaces like the inside of the mouth or vagina, they typically appear as ulcers rather than raised bumps or blisters. Fragile vesicles in soft, damp areas like the labia minora or the area under the foreskin in uncircumcised men are easily broken, leaving painful, shallow ulcers and releasing virus-laden fluid that can spread infection to neighboring areas of skin.

During a primary infection, when the patient has no prior immunity to HSV infection, it is very important that the patient avoid touching his or her lesions. As mentioned earlier, contaminated vesicular fluid can cause infection of the finger (herpetic whitlow) if a break in the epidermis or cuticle is present. A finger moistened with contam-

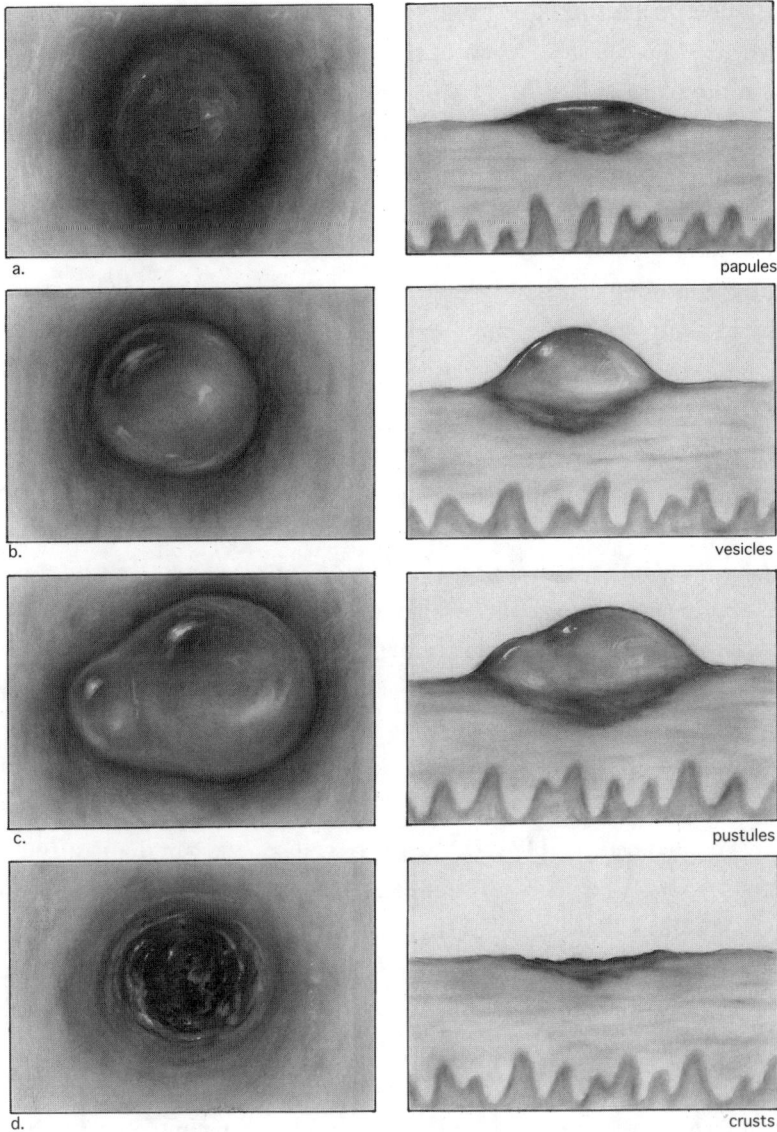

FIGURE 1.61 **Herpes lesion**—(a) Fluid collects at the site of infection, raising the surface of the skin to produce small reddened bumps called **papules.** (b) The continued destruction of neighboring epidermal cells and the collection of additional fluid raises the outermost layer of the epidermis to form delicate, clear bumps or **vesicles,** containing large amounts of infectious HSV. (c) When vesicles rupture, virus in the fluid can spread infection to the surrounding skin. Adjacent vesicles may combine to form **pustules**— larger blisters filled with pus. (d) The blisters form scab-like **crusts** that eventually fall away, and the area heals, usually without leaving a scar.

inated vesicular fluid and brought immediately into contact with one's own face can cause infection of the mouth or eyes. This phenomenon, **autoinoculation,** is unlikely to occur during recurrent episodes of infection because the patient already has antibodies and some degree of acquired immunity to HSV infection.

1.62 Latency, Reactivation, and Recurrence

After initial replication at the original site of infection, HSV is transported along sensory nerves to specialized bundles of nerve cells called **ganglia** where **latency** is established. We use the term "latent" to describe a lingering infection by **dormant** HSV; by "dormant," we mean the HSV is in a slowed-down metabolic state (sort of like a hibernating bear). The terms "latent" and "dormant" are often used interchangeably to describe the "sleeping" virus.

HSV from an initial genital infection travels along the nerves that supply feeling to the genital surface areas and establishes latency where those nerves originate, in the **sacral ganglia** at the base of the spine (see Figure 1.62A). HSV from an initial oral infection is transported along nerves that supply feeling to the mouth and face and establishes latency mainly in the **trigeminal ganglia,** located near the brain stem on the undersurface of the brain (see Figure 1.62B).

The behavior of HSV in the nerve cells of the ganglia is very different from its behavior in skin cells. HSV does not replicate uncontrollably and kill nerve cells. After a brief period of replication to establish itself in the nerve cells, HSV stops replicating and becomes dormant. Periodically, the virus is reactivated, and it travels back along the nerve to the general area of original infection.

Reactivation of dormant HSV is poorly understood. It can occur for no apparent reason or as a result of several known stimuli. Fever, menstruation, poor nutrition, emotional stress, physical exhaustion, trauma to the original site of infection, and exposure to strong ultraviolet light (usually sunburn) are the most frequently noted triggers of reactivation. Much of the time, reactivation causes no lesions, but it does cause a problem: It deposits virus on the surface of the skin or on the mucous membranes. This is called **viral shedding** — sometimes **asymptomatic**

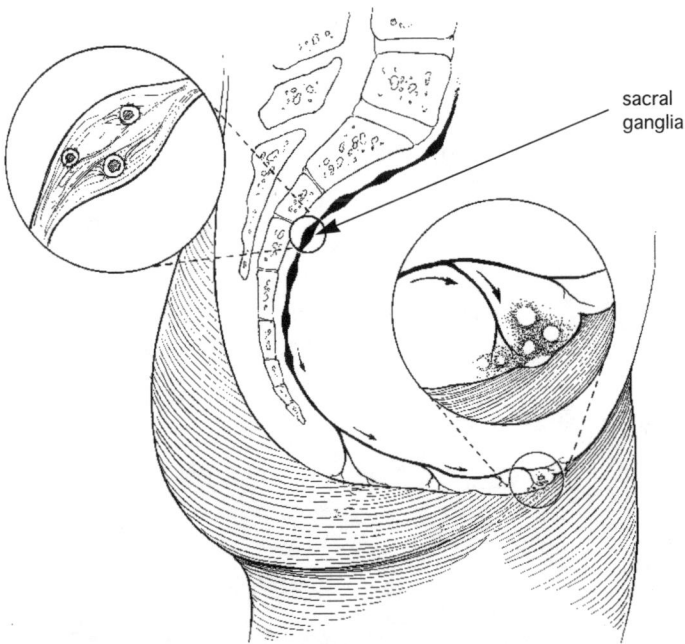

FIGURE 1.62A   The virus responsible for genital herpes lesions remains safe from the immune system inside the nerve roots at the base of the spine called sacral ganglia, shown here in the upper left inset. During reactivation, HSV returns to the skin surface by the same nerve pathways.

viral shedding or **subclinical shedding.** Of course, reactivation is also responsible for the return of herpes lesions and other symptoms, what we term an **outbreak** or a **recurrence.**

The important point is that reactivation, whether it's associated with an outbreak or subclinical shedding, is the first step in the sequence of events that leads to symptoms and the risk of transmission.

1.7 THE ANTIGENIC CONNECTION BETWEEN HSV-1 AND HSV-2

The immune system is our natural defense against infection. We use the term **antigen** to describe any foreign substance, like a bacteria or a virus, that triggers a response by the immune system. Normally, upon detection of a new antigen, specialized white blood cells called B and

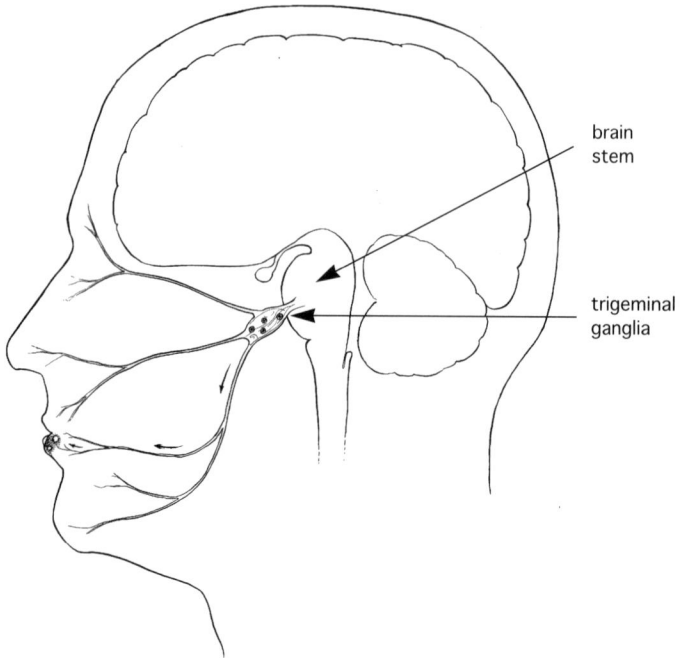

FIGURE 1.62B   Oral herpes infection evades the immune system inside the trigeminal ganglia, at the base of the brain. The connecting nerve pathways serve various sites on the face.

T lymphocytes (the "Marines" of the immune system) spring into action, locating and eliminating the invader.

One of the most remarkable features of the immune system is its capacity for adaptation. Figuratively speaking, the immune system learns to recognize an antigen so it can mobilize a more rapid defensive response if it ever sees that particular antigen again. The first encounter between an antigen and the immune system leads to the production of antigen-specific **antibodies,** which patrol the blood stream after the initial invasion, ready to attack the antigen if it ever returns. We call this acquired protection from infection **immunity.**

HSV-1 and HSV-2 are antigenically distinct versions of herpes simplex virus. They are remarkably similar in structure and composition, more alike than different in most respects. Nonetheless, each provokes its own specific response by the human immune system. We use the term **serotype** to refer to HSV-1 and HSV-2 generically. (The prefix "sero" comes from "serum," the liquid component of blood; antibodies are found in the blood.) When we become infected with either HSV serotype (HSV-1 or HSV-2), the immune system produces serotype-specific antibodies and learns to recognize the invader.

Our immune systems cannot eliminate HSV-1 or HSV-2 completely — *remember, both serotypes establish latent infections that persist for the life of the host* — and we are not protected against recurrent episodes caused by reactivation of dormant virus. We are, however, in almost all cases, immune to reinfection by the same HSV serotype. For example: if you have a history of cold sores, you probably don't have to worry about genital infection by HSV-1. Your cold sores are probably due to latent HSV-1 you acquired years before, and the HSV-1 antibodies in your bloodstream and other immune defenses will probably protect you from developing a second HSV-1 infection at a different anatomic site.

HSV immunity is not absolute. Within both serotype divisions, there are many different **strains** of virus. Strains are unique versions of the virus that differ from each other at the molecular level. Thus, within the serotype of HSV-1, there are many different strains of HSV-1; and within the serotype of HSV-2, there are many different strains of HSV-2. It is *possible, though highly unlikely,* for an otherwise healthy person infected with either HSV-1 or HSV-2 to be reinfected with a different strain of the same serotype. This is a concern primarily in immuno-compromised patients. For all intents and purposes, however, infection with HSV-1 confers immunity to reinfection with HSV-1, and infection with HSV-2 confers immunity to reinfection with HSV-2.

But there's more to this story. HSV-1 and HSV-2 are, as we've noted previously, closely related and very similar — so similar, in fact, that infection with one gives us *partial* immunity to the other. This partial immunity gives us some protection from infection, and reduces the severity of those infections that do occur. Let's consider a hypothetical example:

Two young professionals, George and Eddie — both 25 years old, unmarried, and sexually active. When George was five years old, he had an HSV-1 infection (as do many children), and about once a year, as a result, he gets a cold sore on his lip. Eddie on the other hand, never contracted HSV-1, in any form, at any time. Neither George nor Eddie had ever been infected with HSV-2 until about a year ago when George picked up a woman at a local bar and Eddie went home with a woman he met at a party. Unfortunately, both women had active cases of HSV-2 genital herpes and, shortly after their dangerous liaisons, so did George and Eddie. But there were differences in their symptoms.

George had a few small bumps on either side of the shaft of his penis. As far as he was concerned, it was jock itch, or maybe a rash caused by laundry detergent. It wasn't all that painful, so he didn't even think to see a doctor. In a week or so, it was gone, and in another month, he had forgotten about it altogether.

Eddie, on the other hand, developed a lot of small bumps clustered on the head and shaft of his penis. The bumps spread, became blister-like, and then erupted into extremely painful open sores that eventually crusted over with scabs. Urination was quite painful for Eddie during this initial episode, and for a few days, he discharged a clear fluid from his penis. On top of all that, he had headaches, ran a fever, and felt listless and depressed. His symptoms eventually vanished, just as George's did, but it took about twice as long. Eddie's problems weren't over, however. Two months later, he experienced a recurrence of symptoms. The painful bumps and blisters returned, although they were less numerous and less painful than during the first episode. Now every other month, it's the same story — a recurrent episode of genital herpes — while George has had only a single recurrence of the mysterious rash, which was as unremarkable as the first occurrence.

This example illustrates the role immunity often plays in containing HSV infection. George, who had immunity to HSV-1, still was vulnerable to HSV-2, even from a single sexual encounter with an infected partner. But his immune system was able to respond more quickly than

Eddie's and, hence, do a better job of containing the HSV-2 virus. His first episode was milder than Eddie's, but the HSV-2 virus still infected him, established latency in nerve cells, and recurred. Eddie's immune system, on the other hand, had never seen either HSV serotype and took longer to respond. The HSV-2 virus was able to grow unrestricted for a longer period of time, and he became quite sick as a result. He also suffers from much more severe and frequent recurrences.

In reference to the story above, it is important to note that past infection with HSV-1 doesn't always lessen the severity of an initial HSV-2 infection, nor does it always mollify the severity or frequency of recurrences. Our point here is simply to illustrate the dynamics of partial HSV immunity.

1.8 THE THREE FORMS OF HSV INFECTION

Medically, physicians characterize HSV infection by the site of the infection (mouth, genitals, etc.), the infecting serotype (HSV-1 or HSV-2), and the patient's history of herpes (or lack thereof), as defined by the presence or absence of HSV antibodies in the blood. This history, in turn, defines three forms of infection:

- **Primary**—This is the patient's first HSV infection. The patient has no antibodies to either HSV serotype. Primary infections tend to be the most severe and are the most likely to recur.
- **Nonprimary**—The patient was previously infected by, and now has antibodies to, one HSV serotype, but this is his or her first infection with the other serotype.
- **Recurrent**—The infection was established some time ago, and the current episode is due to reactivation of latent HSV.

In the example of George and Eddie (section 1.7), we would define their infections as follows: Eddie had a primary HSV-2 genital infection because he had no HSV-1 antibodies; George had a nonprimary HSV-2 genital infection because he already had antibodies to HSV-1.

1.9 NONGENITAL HSV INFECTIONS

Our main focus in this book is genital herpes, which can be caused by either HSV-1 or HSV-2. However, both HSV serotypes can also cause a number of nongenital infections — the most common being cold sores or fever blisters on the mouth. Bear in mind that the majority of HSV infections, regardless of the site of infection or the causative HSV serotype, are **asymptomatic** (produce no symptoms). Many nongenital HSV infections are uncommon, but they merit some discussion, especially HSV infections of the eye.

Nongenital HSV infections, including HSV infections of the eye, are profiled in Appendix A.

part
TWO

CYNTHIA'S STORY
Part Two

❧

"Thank you for seeing me on such short notice," Cynthia said, taking a seat in the upholstered armchair across from Dr. Foster's desk in his private office. She sat on the edge of the seat and held her purse on her knees.

Dr. Foster could see she was a little nervous. "That's what we're here for," he said. "I understand you wanted to talk about the vaccine trial here at the Clinic?"

"Maybe," Cynthia said, tentatively. "I don't really know." She began by explaining that two weeks earlier she had been diagnosed with genital herpes. When she saw the ad for the vaccine study in the *Times*, she thought it might be something that could help her. But if nothing else, she hoped at least to get some answers about her infection. She described the intensity of her symptoms and explained that her regular gynecologist told her it was a primary infection. She didn't know what "primary infection" meant, and she couldn't remember most of what Dr. Charles had said at the time because she was so stunned by the news.

"I was supposed to go back for a follow-up visit on Monday," she concluded, "but they canceled the appointment because of an obstetric emergency. They did say the culture was negative—false negative, I think—but I have no idea what that means."

Dr. Foster nodded. "It just means they didn't find any virus growing in the culture. That's not unusual. Dr. Charles is an excellent diagnostician and one of the city's most respected obstetricians. Plus, everything you've said about your symptoms — how you felt and how you responded to antiviral therapy — tells me he was right on the money."

As the conversation continued, Cynthia explained her situation with Brian, how they'd been together four years and had just recently announced their engagement. She confided that she had yet to tell him about the diagnosis and that she had been putting off sex with him by claiming to have a painful yeast infection. "I hate to lie," she said apologetically, "but I just don't feel like I have enough information to talk to him yet, and I was afraid I might still be contagious . . ."

Dr. Foster raised his hand and interrupted gently, "You don't have to explain. You must have been feeling pretty confused. I think you were smart to wait until you had a better grasp of the facts. . . . Did they give you any brochures or other information at Dr. Charles's office?"

Cynthia eased back in the chair and crossed her legs at the ankles. "They did, and I read what they gave me. What I'm hung up on is how I ever got it in the first place. I mean, herpes *is* a venereal disease, right? Like gonorrhea or syphilis?"

Dr. Foster nodded, "We tend to use the term 'sexually transmitted disease' or 'STD' these days, but you're right. Gonorrhea and syphilis are bacterial STDs. Herpes is viral."

Cynthia leaned forward again, squinting slightly. "Is there any way other than sex to catch it? I tried on a bunch of bathing suits on sale at Bloomingdales a few weeks ago. Could I have caught it from that? Or from a toilet seat?"

Dr. Foster smiled and shook his head. "There are some exceptional circumstances that can result in herpes infection of the genitals that do not involve sex, per se, but I don't see that they have any relevance in your case."

Cynthia leaned forward a little further, laying one hand on the front edge of Dr. Foster's desk, "Well, here's what I want to know . . . *one of the things I want to know*. If I haven't had sex with anyone but Brian for the last four years — which I haven't — and if the only way I could have gotten this is from sex . . . " She trailed off, waiting for Dr. Foster to fill in the blank.

"Your reasoning is sound," he said.

"That cheating bastard," Cynthia said in a low tone, sitting back slowly. Then she slammed her fist angrily down against the arm of the chair. "That rotten, lying son-of-a . . ."

Dr. Foster interrupted quickly, shaking his head. "I wouldn't jump to any conclusions. It's entirely possible Brian has had this for years, but not known."

Cynthia looked at him in disbelief. Politely, but with a touch of sarcasm, she said, "Dr. Foster. Excuse me, but I've just been through this, this . . . *hell week* of searing pain and nonstop peeing. . . . How could he *not know?*"

Dr. Foster smiled and nodded. "It's hard to believe, I know. But contrary to your personal experience, *and* popular opinion, genital herpes is usually a very mild disease. At least three-quarters of the people who have it don't know they have it because their symptoms are mild or they have no symptoms at all. It's also an extremely common disease, which is another thing most people don't know. One in every four persons over the age of twelve in this country has genital herpes — at least 45 million people.

"Now, take those two pieces of information and put them together. Fifty million adults with genital herpes — many of them sexually active — and 80 percent of them don't know they're infected. Even when you don't have symptoms — no blisters, no ulcers, no pain — you can still pass the virus on to someone during sex."

"I'm sorry," Cynthia said, shaking her head. "You lost me."

"That's okay," Dr. Foster laughed. "It's a tricky virus and not always easy to understand. Tell you what, let's start at the beginning and," he said, lifting the telephone receiver and punching in some numbers on the keypad, "let's forward this thing so we aren't interrupted." Then he laid the receiver back in its cradle.

"When you were first infected with the herpes virus, some of it got into the nerves that supply feeling to your vagina," Dr. Foster began. "Those nerves are just like a highway or a train track for the virus. It travels back along the length of the nerve to the nerve's point of origin at the base of your spine. Once the virus gets into the nerve cells at the base of your spine, it establishes what we call a "latent" or "dormant" infection. Figuratively speaking, the virus goes to sleep. What did Dr. Charles prescribe for you, anyway?"

"Acyclovir," Cynthia answered. "Acyclovir capsules."

"Okay, while an antiviral drug like acyclovir can be very effective against virus that is replicating in skin tissue and causing painful lesions, it has no effect on dormant virus in the nerve cells at the base of your spine."

"I understand that much." Cynthia said. "It's incurable."

"That's right," Dr. Foster continued. "You have dormant virus *sleeping* in your sacral ganglia, which are little bundles of nerve cells at the base of your spine. And in all probability, every now and then, the virus will reactivate and travel back up the nerves to your genital area . . . "

"And the fun starts all over again," Cynthia sighed, with obvious resignation, setting her purse on the floor beside the chair.

"Well, one of two things happen," Dr. Foster said, smiling, "and this is an oversimplification, but it serves our purposes for the moment. Either you experience another symptomatic outbreak, with lesions that shed infectious virus, *or* you have no signs or symptoms but infectious virus finds its way to the surface of the skin anyway. It's a broad spectrum, actually. You could have anything from excruciatingly painful lesions, to a few little bumps that you never even notice, to zero symptoms altogether. The point is, that even in the absence of symptoms, you could periodically have infectious herpes virus on your genital surfaces and pass the disease on to someone else during sex. This could explain what happened between you and Brian. His dormant herpes virus reawakened. It traveled up a nerve to his penis and reproduced in the skin cells there. The virus worked its way to the surface of the skin and was deposited on your vaginal surfaces during intercourse, even though he never experienced any symptoms." Dr. Foster stopped and raised his eyebrows. "Am I going too fast?"

"No, no. Go on."

"Well this is my conclusion, based on what you've said so far. In my opinion, you caught genital herpes from Brian. That doesn't mean he cheated on you *or* that he didn't. But considering the seriousness of your relationship and all the plans you two have made, I'd give him the benefit of a doubt."

Cynthia was still skeptical, "I understand how this is *possible,* but how common is it?"

"It's just an estimate," Dr. Foster said, "but we're pretty sure about seventy percent of new cases of genital herpes are the result of asymptomatic viral shedding. And one more thing, before we go any further—based on what you've told me, I'd have to say that you two *probably* aren't eligible for the current vaccine study. It's for couples in which only one partner is infected. I'm pretty sure if we gave Brian a blood test, it would tell us that he's already infected."

Cynthia seemed to have accepted Dr. Foster's explanation, albeit hesitantly. "There's still the question of when he got this asymptomatic infection," she said.

Dr. Foster opened his hands, turned his palms upward, and shrugged his shoulders.

Cynthia continued, "If he's had it all this time, why, after four years, did I finally catch it? Why not the year before, or the year before that?"

"Who knows?" Dr. Foster said, shaking his head. "Chance. Bad luck. Whatever. Statistics say the risk of transmission in a couple is about ten percent per year. I've seen couples in which one partner—the man, say—has had symptomatic genital herpes for eight or nine years. They're as sexually active as the next couple, but for some reason, the woman has never contracted it. In other cases, within a year or two, both partners are infected despite the precautions of condoms and abstinence during symptomatic outbreaks."

Cynthia had calmed down completely since her brief outburst of fist-pounding rage. "There's another thing that's been bothering me, if you have the time," she said.

Dr. Foster glanced at his watch. "Plenty of time. Go ahead."

"I'm concerned about having sex with Brian now. Should I be worried about giving it back to him?"

"Reinfecting him with the same virus he gave you?" Dr. Foster asked. "Not unless he has weakened immunity in some way."

Cynthia looked around the room. She seemed to be weighing the import of this last bit of information. Then she shifted in her chair and looked Dr. Foster squarely in the eye. In a slightly conspiratorial tone, she asked, "If there's no danger of Brian getting herpes from me — *obviously, he's already got it*— then I guess I could just keep all this to myself, *couldn't I?* I mean, why bring it up?"

Dr. Foster took a deep breath, and leaned forward slightly, "Well," he said, "that's your decision, of course. It's not my place to make that kind of judgment, but you might want to consider the potential for Brian to do harm to others. Remote as the chances may be, if Brian ever were unfaithful to you, or for some reason you two ever split up, my concern as a physician is that Brian might pass this disease on to yet another woman . . . or women."

"What if *I'm* the one who's had it for years," Cynthia said, "and this is just the first time it has showed up in me. How can you be so sure?"

"That's an insightful thought," Dr. Foster said enthusiastically. "Theoretically, yes — you could have experienced the first symptomatic recurrence of a latent infection you've had since who knows when. But the intensity of your symptoms points to a primary first episode, not a recurrence. And we have the strength of Dr. Charles's opinion to back us up on that."

Dr. Foster made a couple of notes on the yellow legal pad on the desk before him. Then he lay his pen down and leaned back in his chair, "By any chance," he asked, "did they draw blood for serologic testing at Dr. Charles's office?"

Cynthia shrugged, "The nurse took some blood. She didn't say what for."

"Did you reschedule your follow-up visit?"

"Next Friday."

"When you talk to Dr. Charles, ask him if he ordered a type-specific serology, like a Western blot." Dr. Foster wrote "Type-specific serology? Results?" on a page in the legal pad, tore it out, and slid it across the desk to Cynthia. "There are two kinds of herpes simplex virus.

HSV-1 is the virus most often associated with cold sores. HSV-2 is the one that's usually responsible for genital herpes. Primary infection with HSV-2, which is what we think you probably had, occurs when the host—*that's you*—was not previously infected with either virus type. Do you have any history of cold sores?"

Cynthia shook her head. "None that I can remember."

"So there y'go. Now, if Dr. Charles ordered a blood test and it came back negative for both virus types, that would confirm the diagnosis of primary infection. What did they tell you when they called to cancel your original follow-up?"

"The nurse said all the tests were negative, but I thought she was just talking about the viral culture. I'll ask on Friday."

"If we to were to test you now," Dr. Foster said, "or maybe in a couple more weeks just to be on the safe side, I bet we'd find you have no antibodies to HSV-1, just antibodies to HSV-2 from your recent infection. It wouldn't be a bad idea for Brian to get tested, by the way. If you decide to tell him."

"Oh, I'm going to tell him," Cynthia said. "I think it's the right thing to do."

"It's a good idea," Dr. Foster agreed, "for a lot of different reasons. But let me caution you, initially, Brian may reject the news. No one wants genital herpes. Remember what an awful shock it was for you? And you were already at the gynecologist's office complaining of intense vaginal pain. He's going to hear this out of the clear blue from the woman he loves, his fiancée no less. That's got to be a shock. He may need some time to absorb the blow and recover.

"We still don't know if you had a blood test at Dr. Charles's office, but if you did, and if it was negative for both virus types, I would recommend you be tested again in another couple of weeks. That will remove any lingering doubt in your mind that you actually have herpes. It could also confirm that yours was a primary episode and that you acquired the infection from Brian. Testing is probably a good idea for him, too. He may have a hard time accepting the fact that he has genital herpes, if there's no physical evidence."

"Oh, perfect," Cynthia laughed.

"What?" Dr. Foster asked smiling.

"'Physical evidence.' *Brian's a lawyer.*"

～

In the time remaining, Dr. Foster answered more of Cynthia's questions and explained her therapeutic options for recurrent episodes of infection. As she was preparing to leave, she asked whether he was taking new patients and whether he thought Dr. Charles would mind if she transferred her gynecological care to the Women's Clinic.

"That's completely up to you," he said. "You should do what you want to do. It's your body and your health. But I don't think his feelings would be hurt, if that's your concern. He runs a busy practice up there. But do go for that follow-up, and be sure to ask about the type-specific blood test."

As Cynthia rose from her chair, Dr. Foster also stood. They shook hands, and she said, "Well I think I'm going to come here from now on. And tonight, I'm going to tell Brian about all this."

chapter two

GENITAL HERPES:
FACTS AND FIGURES

∾

2.1 THE ONGOING EPIDEMIC: A BRIEF HISTORY

Up until the late 1970s and early 1980s, most people in America had never heard of genital herpes. Then, out of the clear blue, it was front-page news. Physicians were reporting a dramatic rise in the number of patients with severe disease that took weeks to resolve and returned periodically. There was no cure and no effective treatment to ease the symptoms. Most patients were young middle-class whites — so much so that in some circles, genital herpes was actually known as "the VD of the Ivy League."

Genital herpes also seemed to appear out of nowhere at the height of the sexual revolution, and it quickly became stigmatized in the public mind as a sign of promiscuity and moral decline. Some saw in it a sort of divine retribution. Some jokingly referred to it as Jerry Falwell's revenge. In 1980, *Time* magazine characterized genital herpes as "the new sexual leprosy" and, in a now legendary 1982 cover story, proclaimed the emergence of "The New Scarlet Letter." Such negative associations persist today, which is unfortunate because they have absolutely nothing to do with the reality of the disease.

No one really understood genital herpes 15 or 20 years ago, not even the medical profession. At that time, genital herpes was wrongly characterized as a relatively rare and usually severe disease. But actually, what we were seeing in the early 1980s was a significant increase in **primary genital herpes,** which tends to be the most severe form of infection. Patients with severe symptoms were seeking help from doctors; patients with mild disease were not. And physicians were describing the disease to the American public based on the cases they were treating at the time. Accordingly, people were not told that herpes could also cause mild symptoms. Of course, we now know that the vast majority of people with genital herpes have disease so mild they aren't even aware they are infected. We've also learned that genital herpes is very common.

Let's pause a moment and review some of our terminology.

- **Symptomatic vs. asymptomatic**—A significant percentage of HSV-2 infections are asymptomatic: they cause no obvious signs or symptoms (no rash, no sores, no swollen glands, etc.), so the infected person doesn't know he or she has genital herpes. The term "unrecognized" also comes into play, in that herpes often causes symptoms so mild that they may be unrecognized by someone who isn't looking for them. Up to 80 percent of people with genital herpes have either asymptomatic or unrecognized infection.
- **Primary vs. nonprimary**—In section 1.7 we learned that HSV-1 and HSV-2 are so similar in their make-up that infection with one gives us partial immunity to the other. For example: infection with HSV-1 confers partial immunity to infection with HSV-2. While this partial immunity may not protect us from HSV-2 infection completely, it tends to lessen the severity of the initial HSV-2 infection and to reduce the likelihood and frequency of recurrences. When partial immunity is in force, the initial episode of infection is called *nonprimary*. A *primary* infection occurs when we have no immunity. Primary infections, when symptomatic, are generally more severe, longer-lasting, and more likely to recur than nonprimary infections.

How do we account for the historic increase in primary HSV-2 infection back in the late '70s and early '80s? The putative explanation is that an increasing number of Americans were reaching young adulthood and becoming sexually active without ever becoming infected with HSV-1—a change attributed largely to a rising standard of living. This answer is consistent with the epidemiologic data. Until relatively recent years, virtually everyone in America was infected with HSV-1 by the time they reached puberty. In other words, just about everyone had partial immunity to HSV-2. HSV-2 infection, when it occurred, tended to be mild or asymptomatic; recurrent infections were less common; and genital herpes was largely unrecognized and rarely suspected as a sexually transmitted disease.

Today, however, the prevalence of HSV-1 infection among young white adults is estimated to have fallen to between 50 and 60 percent. While this change in the rate of primary HSV-1 infection may explain the increase in primary HSV-2 infection among middle-class whites in the late '70s and early '80s, it alone cannot account for the overall increase in genital herpes. Other factors cited as causes of the current epidemic include a general increase in sexual activity in the 1960s and 1970s (the so-called sexual revolution); declining fear of "older" STDs like gonorrhea and syphilis, which are easily cured with modern antibiotics; changes in lifestyle (people starting to have sex earlier, remaining single longer, divorcing more readily and more often); and the declining use of barrier contraceptives, particularly condoms, with the advent of the birth control pill.

2.2 EPIDEMIOLOGY

Epidemiology is the branch of medicine that studies, among other things, the distribution of diseases in the population. Epidemiologists use two basic terms to describe the distribution of disease: "prevalence" and "incidence." **Prevalence** is the total number of people who have a particular disease at any given point in time. It can be expressed in terms of geographic area (city, state, country, etc.) or demographic group (men, women, children, elderly, blacks, whites, etc.). **Incidence,** on the other hand, is the number of new cases occurring in a given time period, usually *per year,* and can likewise be applied to any geographic or demographic subgroup. In the case of genital herpes, we can also describe its prevalence and incidence according to causative serotype, either HSV-1 or HSV-2.

2.21 HSV-1 or HSV-2?

Between 85 and 95 percent of existing (prevalent) cases of genital herpes are caused by HSV-2. However, somewhere between 10 and 50 percent of new (incident) cases are caused by HSV-1. This increase in genital HSV-1 infection is due mainly to two factors: 1.) In general, oral-genital sexual behavior has increased in recent decades; and 2.) More people today are becoming sexually active without ever having been infected with HSV-1.

2.22 Incidence and Prevalence of Genital Herpes

Because we don't hear as much about genital herpes today as we did back in the early 1980s, many people mistakenly believe it has become less common. Nothing could be further from the truth. Genital herpes is a very common disease. It has been estimated that roughly one million individuals in the United States are newly infected each year.

According to a major study recently published in the *New England Journal of Medicine,* roughly 45 million people in the United States have type 2 genital herpes —26 percent of women 12 years of age or older and 18 percent of men in the same age group (Fleming 1997). These estimates are based on data from the third National Health and Nutrition Examination Survey (NHANES III), a federally funded research project that includes taking blood samples for testing from a cross-section of the U.S. population. The previous genital herpes prevalence estimate of 16.4 percent, overall, was based on NHANES II samples collected between 1976 and 1980. The latest estimate, based on samples collected from 1988 to 1994, shows that, in the interim, *the prevalence of genital herpes increased by more than 30 percent!* The greatest increases were seen among young whites — a five-fold increase among white teenagers and a two-fold increase among whites in their twenties. Data from NHANES II and III, broken down by sex and major ethnic subgroup, are summarized in Table 2.22.

It's worth noting that the 30 percent increase in genital herpes occurred during the rise of AIDS, a time when more and more people were presumably practicing "safer sex." This tells us something, perhaps, about the inefficiency of condoms in preventing the spread of genital herpes — a topic we will return to later. It may also indicate that despite the AIDS epidemic, many sexually active people did not use condoms in the 1980s.

TABLE 2.22   PERCENTAGE OF NHANES II AND NHANES III SUBJECTS WITH HSV-2 ANTIBODIES, BY SEX AND MAJOR ETHNIC GROUP*

	NHANES II (1976–1980) % positive for HSV-2	NHANES III (1988–1994) % positive for HSV-2	Percent increase
ALL SUBJECTS			
Both sexes	16	21	30
Men	13	17	27
Women	18	24	32
WHITES			
Both sexes	13	17	30
Men	11	14	32
Women	15	19	29
BLACKS			
Both sexes	44	48	9
Men	34	38	10
Women	51	56	8

(Fleming 1997)

* HSV-2 seroprevalence (the percentage of population positive for HSV-2 antibodies) has been age-adjusted to the 1980 census. The age range is 12 years or older.

2.3 Transmission

Most people think, "If I had herpes, I'd know." Unfortunately, that's just not true. In fact, the spread of genital herpes is greatly facilitated by the fact that most people have mild or asymptomatic cases and are not aware they carry the disease. However, an interesting study at the University of Washington in Seattle (Langenburg 1995) showed that about half of patients who have genital herpes and don't know it can identify a recurrent episode within 12 months of being trained to recognize the signs and symptoms.

If we could just find a way to identify asymptomatic patients and train them to recognize their own recurrent infections, we might go a long way toward reducing the current epidemic.

At present, we are teaching physicians and patients to suspect HSV infection whenever recurrent lesions are part of the clinical picture, no matter how mild — including recurrent lesions on the anus, thighs, and buttocks, not just the genitals. In fact, roughly 10 percent of men and 30 percent of women with herpes experience lesions on the buttocks or thighs.

Regarding transmission, a question on the minds of most people with genital herpes is, *"What is the risk to my partner?"* This issue has been studied in discordant heterosexual couples. When we speak of **discordant** couples in reference to genital herpes, we don't mean couples who argue. We are referring to couples in which one partner has genital herpes and the other does not.

According to one study, the average risk of transmission in discordant couples is about 10 percent per year. Theoretically, this means if we started the year with 1,000 discordant couples in which only one partner was infected, at the end of one year, both partners in 100 of those couples would have genital herpes, and 900 would remain discordant. After another year, both partners in 90 more couples would be infected; 810 would remain discordant, etc. With each passing year, the number of discordant couples would decrease by 10 percent. However (and this is a big "however"), 10 percent is an average; it does not take into account which member of the couple was originally infected, nor does it reflect the gender-specific differences in risk. It appears that the annual risk for a woman in discordant couples is twice as high as it is for a man. This means that a woman with an HSV-2–positive male partner may have a 15 percent chance of getting genital herpes in one year, while a man with an HSV-2–positive female partner may have only a 4 to 8 percent chance. This discrepancy mirrors the fact that women are generally at greater risk for genital herpes than men.

2.4 RISK FACTORS

When doctors speak of risk factors for a particular disease they mean human traits, behaviors, and circumstances that increase a person's chance of having that disease. In the case of genital herpes, eight main risk factors have been identified.

1. **Age at first sexual intercourse.** The earlier you begin to engage in sexual intercourse, presuming you will continue to have intercourse in the years that follow, the more likely you are to have sex with a person who has an active HSV-2 infection, and the more likely you are to catch genital herpes. Knowledge of safer sex practices and appreciation for the risks involved in sexual activities are also presumed to be less developed in the young.

2. **Number of sexual partners.** This is common sense. The more people you have sex with, the more likely you are to have sex with someone who has an active HSV-2 infection and catch genital herpes.

3. **Gender.** A woman's risk of getting genital herpes is substantially greater than a man's, for three possible reasons: First, women have a larger susceptible area for infection — the entire mucocutaneous surface area of the vagina and cervix and the moist, delicate, enfolded tissues of the labia minora. Second, women typically receive and retain a larger quantity of virus per sexual encounter. And third, many young women have sex with older men, who are more likely to have acquired HSV-2.

An important note: In addition to being at greater risk for acquisition of HSV-2, women are at greater risk for all STDs. They generally have more complications from STDs, and the complications are more likely to be severe, long-lasting, or permanent (e.g., infertility, ectopic pregnancy, cervical cancer, and sick babies). It is critically important for women who are diagnosed with any STD, including genital herpes, to be tested for other STDs as well. See Item 4, below.

4. **History of other sexually transmitted disease (STD).** If you have ever had gonorrhea, syphilis, or another STD, you are more likely to have acquired an HSV-2 infection than someone with no STD history. If you have sexual contact with a person who has had one of these diseases, you are also at increased risk for genital herpes. Why? Acquisition of an STD suggests high-risk behavior (unprotected sex). In addition, some STDs tend to produce lesions — sores, ulcers, and other breaches in the skin of the genitals and surrounding areas. These lesions can be portals of entry for other viruses, bacteria, and fungi. By the same token, a history of genital herpes is a risk factor for the acquisition of other STDs, including AIDS. If your doctor suspects you have genital herpes, it's part of the recommended work-up to test you for several other STDs as well. If you have been diagnosed with genital herpes but were not tested for other STDs, you should be. If your doctor says it isn't necessary, find another doctor, or go to a local STD clinic for testing. It's simple, it's good medicine, and it's good public health policy. Plus it's always in your best interest to know the truth about your state of sexual health.

5. **Low family income.** The prevalence and incidence of virtually every infectious disease is inversely related to socioeconomic status. This is not a value judgment. People of low income have less access to educational and health care resources.

6. **Increasing number of years of sexual activity.** Again, this is common sense. The risk of HSV-2 infection rises with increasing sexual exposure. Outside the context of long-term monogamous relationships, the more years you are sexually active, the more people you will have sex with, and the greater will be your chance of contracting genital herpes.

7. **Age.** More than 80 percent of all primary genital herpes occurs in those aged 15–35.

8. **Race.** There are no known differences in racial susceptibility to HSV infection. Overall, the greatest increase in genital herpes in the United States between 1988 and 1994 was in the white population. The prevalence of HSV-2 infection is roughly three times higher among blacks than whites. Earlier age at first intercourse is a likely contributing factor along with the fact that once the prevalence is high in a population, the likelihood of contact with the virus will remain high.

In Table 2.4, we see the reality of some of these and other risk factors reflected in data from the most recent NHANES report (Fleming 1997).

2.5 SYMPTOMS

About 80 percent of all HSV infections (primary, nonprimary, and recurrent) produce no symptoms; or symptoms are so mild they're easily mistaken for something else, like eczema, heat rash, jock itch, a pimple, or an ingrown hair. Symptomatic primary infections tend to be the most severe and the longest-lasting; recurrent infections tend to be the mildest; and nonprimary infections lie somewhere in between.

The first time a person notes the symptoms related to herpes may be years after he or she first acquired the virus. Up to 25 percent of reported first episodes of infection are actually the first symptomatic recurrence of a previously silent infection.

Table 2.4   HSV-2 Infection by Selected Demographic and Behavioral Characteristics—NHANES III*

Characteristic	Percent of subjects infected with HSV-2
MARITAL STATUS	
Single	17
Married	22
Divorced or separated	39
Widowed	35
EDUCATION (LAST YEAR COMPLETED)	
Elementary	35
High school	24
Some college	19
RESIDENCE	
Urban	23
Nonurban	21
ECONOMIC STATUS	
Below poverty level	34
At or above poverty level	21
EVER USED COCAINE	
Yes	34
No	21
AGE AT FIRST INTERCOURSE (YRS)	
17 or younger	27
18 or older	19
LIFETIME NUMBER OF SEX PARTNERS	
0	3
1	10
2–4	21
5–9	26
10–49	31
50 or more	46

(Fleming 1997)

*National Health and Nutrition Examination Survey (1988–1994)

2.51 Symptomatic Primary Genital Herpes*

Primary genital herpes infections caused by HSV-1 tend to be just as severe and long-lasting as those caused by HSV-2, but they are less likely to recur. On average, the time between sexual contact and the first appearance of symptoms is 3 to 7 days, but it may be as short as 1 day or may exceed 14 days.

WOMEN

Symptomatic primary genital herpes is generally more severe in women than in men. It may start with a short period of itching, burning, tenderness, and redness in the area around the labia minora and the vaginal opening. Vesicles (clear, dome-shaped blisters) may then appear on the labia minora, labia majora, and other areas in and around the vaginal opening. The distribution of lesions tends to be bilateral (left and right). New lesions (vesicles) may continue to appear and spread to neighboring areas, including the thighs, buttocks, and anal region. (See Figure 2.51A.)

Vesicles on soft, moist external tissues like the labia minora tend to rupture soon after they appear, leaving painful ulcers (shallow depressions in the skin) that are covered with yellowish-gray pus-like fluid and surrounded by a distinct halo of reddened skin. On drier surfaces, like the skin of the thighs and buttocks, vesicles tend to remain intact, fill with pus, and then dry out, leaving a crust or scab. Mucosal lesions generally have an ulcer-like appearance.

Vesicles continue to appear for seven days or more. Clusters of vesicles may coalesce to form larger lesions, progressing to extensive areas of ulceration that resemble second-degree burns. The cervix usually becomes infected, and a watery vaginal discharge is not uncommon. The external genitalia will be painful when touched. Inflammation of the urethra almost always occurs, and dysuria (painful urination) may be bad enough to cause urinary retention (holding in of urine).

---

* First episode of symptomatic infection, and the patient has no antibodies to HSV-1 or HSV-2

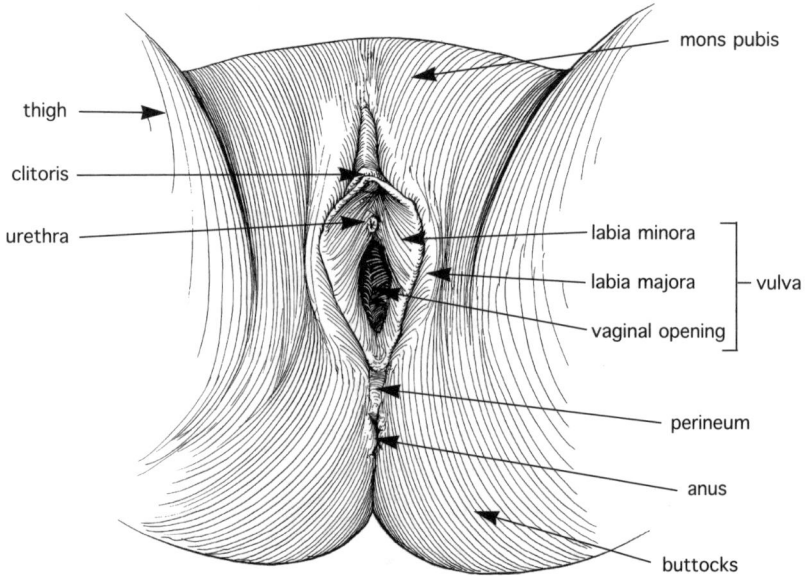

FIGURE 2.51A Herpes lesions in women may be located anywhere in the genital region, most frequently on the vulva.

Most women with primary symptomatic genital herpes will have **constitutional symptoms** in addition to the **local symptoms** described above (those localized to the site of infection). Constitutional symptoms include fever, headache, malaise (a vague feeling of bodily discomfort), muscle aches, and loss of appetite. Most women will also have painful swollen lymph nodes in the groin and pelvic areas.

Constitutional symptoms usually last three to four days and disappear toward the end of the first week. Local symptoms usually intensify through the first seven days, peak between days eight and ten, then gradually subside. Pain is usually gone in 10 to 14 days. Lesions heal, usually without scarring, in two to four weeks. Viral replication is greatest around days three and four. It usually lasts 11 to 12 days, but may continue from the cervix for several weeks, even after external lesions have healed.

MEN

Lesions can appear on both sides of the glans (head or tip), foreskin, and shaft of the penis. Lesions on the scrotum, thighs and buttocks are less common. (See Figure 2.51B.) The course of lesion formation in men is similar to that in women. Most men will have pain, itching, swelling, and inflammation in the affected areas. Difficult urination and a clear fluid discharged from the penis are seen in 30 to 40 percent of cases. Men may also have swollen lymph nodes in the groin and pelvic regions, but this constitutional symptom is usually more severe in women. Less than 50 percent of men with primary symptomatic genital herpes have significant constitutional symptoms. Viral shedding is at its peak during days three to five and lasts for about 10 to 11 days. Pain is usually gone by the end of week two, and healing of lesions without scarring can be expected in two to three weeks.

Table 2.51 shows the average frequency and duration of signs and symptoms of primary genital HSV-2 infection in men and women treated

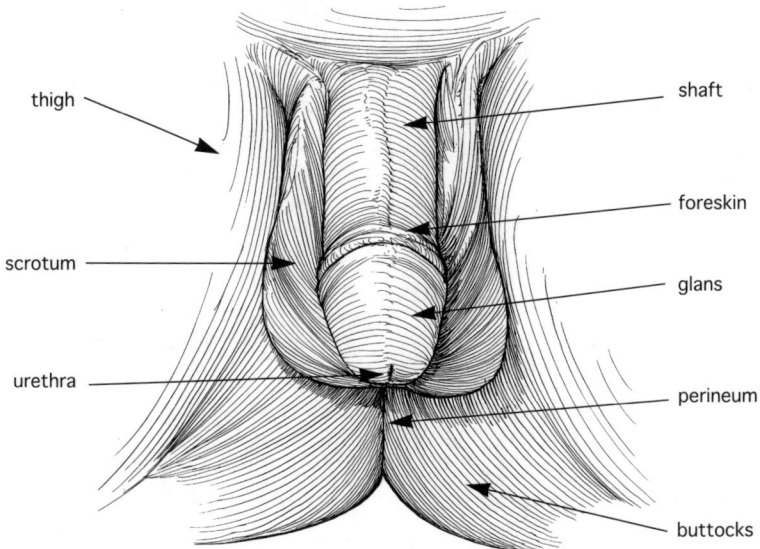

FIGURE 2.51B Herpes lesions in men may be located anywhere in the genital region, though they are seldom found on the glans of the penis.

Table 2.51 Selected Clinical Characteristics of Patients during a Primary Symptomatic Episode of Genital HSV-2 Infection

	Men	Women
Constitutional symptoms (fever, headache, malaise, muscle pain)	39%	68%
Meningitis (see Section 1.84)	11%	36%
Pain at the site of infection (genital pain)	95%	99%
Average duration of genital pain	10.9 days	11.9 days
Dysuria (painful or difficult urination)	44%	83%
Average duration of dysuria	7.2 days	11.9 days
Urethral or vaginal discharge	27%	85%
Average duration of discharge	5.6 days	12.9 days
Tender adenopathy (swollen lymph nodes)	80%	81%
Average duration of tender adenopathy	8.6 days	14.2 days
Average total surface area of genital lesions	427 mm²	550 mm²
Average duration of viral shedding from lesions	10.5 days	11.8 days
HSV-2 cultured from the urethra	28%	76%
HSV-2 cultured from the cervix	—	88%
Average duration of cervical shedding	—	11.4 days
Average time for lesions to heal	16.5 days	19.7 days

(Corey 1990)

at the University of Washington Genital HSV Clinic. The data indicate that women tend to have more severe and longer-lasting symptoms.

2.52 Symptomatic Nonprimary Genital Herpes*

The symptoms of nonprimary genital herpes are similar to those of primary infection, but they tend to be less severe and of shorter duration. Among other differences, constitutional symptoms, extragenital lesions (on the legs and buttocks), and complications are less common in nonprimary infection, and lesions on mucous membranes are rare. Women

---

* First episode of symptomatic infection, but the patient has antibodies to the noninfecting HSV serotype

TABLE 2.52 SELECTED CLINICAL CHARACTERISTICS OF
PATIENTS WITH SYMPTOMATIC PRIMARY AND
NONPRIMARY GENITAL HSV-2 INFECTION

	Primary	Nonprimary
Constitutional symptoms		
(fever, headache, malaise, muscle pain)	62%	16%
Average duration of genital pain	11.8 days	8.7 days
Average number of lesions	15.5	9.5
Lesions formed on left and right side of		
genitals	82%	55%
New lesions formed after infection was		
underway	75%	45%
Average duration of viral shedding from lesions	11.4 days	6.8 days
Average time for lesions to heal	18.6 days	15.5 days
(Corey 1990)		

are less likely to shed virus from the cervix during a nonprimary infection. Table 2.52 illustrates some of the differences between primary and nonprimary HSV-2 genital herpes.

2.53 Symptomatic Recurrent Genital Herpes

As a rule, the more severe the initial infection, the more severe the recurrent infection, but overall, recurrent genital herpes tends to be less severe and of shorter duration than the original episode. And remember: The majority of people with genital herpes actually have mild symptoms or none at all. Up to 90 percent who have antibodies to HSV-2 give no history of the disease when interviewed.

Among those who have recognized HSV, recurrences often appear at the site of the original infection. However, since the ganglia where HSV establishes latency innervate a wide region of the genital area, recurrent lesions on the thighs and buttocks are also common. Lesions typically begin as a cluster of small reddened bumps and evolve into clear vesicles on a base of reddened skin, the appearance of which has been compared to dew drops on a rose petal. The vesicles break open and may evolve into ulcerations. The course of lesion formation is similar to that seen in primary and nonprimary episodes, but the area of involvement tends to be smaller. Recurrent infections produce fewer and less painful lesions, and the lesions tend to be concentrated on one or the other side of the affected area or organ, as opposed to the bilateral distribution characteristic of primary and nonprimary infection.

Recurrent infection produces more severe symptoms in women than in men. Lesions usually appear on the labia minora, labia majora, and perineum but may also form on the mons pubis, perianal area, and buttocks. (See illustration, page 58.) Swollen lymph nodes are reported by some women, but fever and constitutional symptoms are rare. Pain usually resolves by the end of the first week, and lesions disappear in eight to ten days.

In men, symptomatic recurrence usually produces a patch of grouped vesicles on one side of the glans, foreskin, or shaft of the penis, but these may also form on the scrotum, perianal area, thighs and buttocks. (See illustration, page 59.) These vesicles follow a typical course to crusting, as described in previous sections. Sixty percent of men report pain during recurrent episodes, but constitutional symptoms are rare. Viral shedding is usually less intense and of shorter duration, and lesions heal in seven to ten days.

Table 2.53 shows the average frequency and duration of signs and symptoms of recurrent genital HSV-2 infection in men and women treated at the University of Washington Genital HSV Clinic. However, it should be noted that these data, gathered in the 1980s, were collected from patients with disease severe enough to drive them to the clinic for treatment (i.e., their symptoms were generally more severe than those experienced by the majority of people with herpes).

2.54 Prodromal Symptoms

Most people with recurrent genital herpes experience a phenomenon known as a **prodrome.** The prodrome is a collection of variable symptoms that appear anywhere from a couple of hours to a couple of days before a recurrent episode of infection. Each person's prodrome is unique,

TABLE 2.53   SELECTED CLINICAL CHARACTERISTICS OF
PATIENTS WITH RECURRENT GENITAL HSV-2 INFECTION

	Men	*Women*
Prodromal symptoms	53%	43%
Average number of lesions at onset of episode	7.5	4.8
Lesion pain	67%	88%
Average duration of lesion pain	3.9 days	5.9 days
Average total surface area of genital lesions	62.7 mm^2	53.5 mm^2
Lesions on left and right sides of genitals	15%	4%
New lesions formed after episode was underway	43%	28%
Average duration of new lesion formation	5.2 days	5.4 days
Lesions present at nongenital sites	3%	5%
Itching at genital sites	85%	87%
Average duration of itching	4.6 days	5.2 days
Dysuria (painful or difficult urination)	9%	27%
Urethral or vaginal discharge	4%	45%
Average duration of discharge	1.7 days	5.3 days
Tender adenopathy (swollen lymph nodes)	23%	31%
Average duration of tender adenopathy	9.2 days	5.9 days
HSV-2 cultured from the cervix	—	12%
Average duration of cervical shedding	—	3.2 days
Average time to crusting (scabbing) of lesions	4.1 days	4.7 days
Average time for lesions to heal	10.6 days	9.3 days
Average duration of viral shedding from lesions	4.4 days	4.1 days
(Corey 1990)		

but among the symptoms that have been reported are pain, itching, tingling, burning, or tenderness at the site of the original infection. Some patients report sudden shooting pains that follow the path of one or more nerves in the back and are confined to the same side of the body that becomes the focus of lesions. This back pain may be accompanied by severe burning, aching, or shooting pains in the leg, buttock, or genital area.

In some cases, prodromal symptoms are the only symptoms the person experiences. This is an important point because it means a person can be alerted to the likelihood that he or she is infectious and shedding virus even when no lesions are evident by self-examination. Learning to recognize one's own prodrome is also a key step in the management of genital herpes; one important mode of drug therapy depends on the patient's ability to tell when a recurrent infection is on the way. Medication can abort an outbreak, and the earlier it is started, the better its chance of working.

2.6 Patterns of Recurrence

Genital herpes can arrive undetected, hide in the body for years, and then appear without warning. Most of what we know about recurrence rates is derived from the follow-up of patients with symptomatic first episodes — primary and nonprimary. Based on this, researchers feel they have a good idea of the probability and frequency of recurrence in the population at large, though it really isn't possible to predict what any given individual's experience will be. That said, the following generalizations, estimates, and averages will help you better understand:

- About 90 percent of people with symptomatic first episodes due to HSV-2 have recurrences in the following year: 38 percent will have six or more recurrences; 20 percent will have more than ten.
- HSV-1 is less likely to recur than HSV-2. About 50 percent of persons with genital HSV-1 infection will have a recurrence in the first 12 months after initial infection. The average recurrence rate for HSV-2 is about four episodes per year.
- In the first year after a symptomatic primary HSV-2 infection, men have about 20 percent more recurrences than women.
- The use of antiviral drug therapy to treat the primary infection has no effect on recurrence rate but can dramatically reduce the frequency and severity of recurrences when used on a daily basis thereafter.

2.7 DIAGNOSIS: WHAT TO EXPECT, WHAT TO DEMAND

2.71 A Complete History

If you find yourself seeking medical attention for what seems to be an STD, your doctor will need to take a thorough medical history. A history is precisely what it sounds like: a record of important past events — injuries, diseases, symptoms, treatments — and relevant background on your lifestyle and your family. In addition to the usual questions about your personal health and family medical history, you should be asked about any past or recurring medical problems involving your genitals and urinary tract. You should expect to be asked about your patterns of sexual activity, your past and present partners, and the use of recreational drugs (including alcohol), which tend to impair one's judgment in sexual situations and increase the likelihood of high-risk behavior, such as unprotected sex.

Most of us prefer to keep our sex life private, and many doctors find these questions as embarrassing to ask as you may find them embarrassing to answer. But be prepared, and try to relax. Remember: the history plays an important role in guiding the diagnostic process. The more accurate and detailed the history, the more likely your doctor is to make an accurate diagnosis and offer useful advice.

Standard operating procedures vary from one doctor's office to another. But the history should always precede the examination, and you should not be required to discuss your sex life while seated on an examination table wearing nothing but a thin paper gown. Many people tend to feel more vulnerable and defensive under those circumstances and are, therefore, less likely to be open and communicative about the intimate details of their lives. If you feel uncomfortable with the circumstances under which the interview is proceeding, express your feelings. It's important to find a way to discuss these issues that puts you both at ease, but try to keep in mind that your doctor needs the information to make the right diagnostic assumptions and provide the best level of care.

2.72 Physical Examination

In addition to taking a sexual history, your doctor will need to perform a thorough examination, including visual examination of the genital area. For women, this will also mean visual inspection of the cervix. Genital herpes accounts for about two-thirds of all genital ulcer disease treated in STD clinics in the United States. So if you arrive at your doctor's office with a genital complaint and you have herpes-like lesions in the genital area, the prime suspect is going to be genital herpes. However, visual examination is only one part of a complete diagnostic work-up. For one thing, genital herpes doesn't look the same in every patient; it can "mimic" the appearance of other STDs, and other STDs can mimic herpes. A mild case of herpes can easily be mistaken for something as innocuous as a pimple, an ingrown hair, or a simple rash. Your doctor will order a laboratory test for herpes, but it may still be necessary to test you for other specific STDs. If a genital lesion is present, you should expect and request that the doctor perform a **viral culture** or some other HSV-specific test. Clinical diagnosis based on visual examination alone is not sufficient.

2.73 Testing for HSV

Viral culture. The "gold standard" of laboratory testing for HSV is a technique called viral culture. It is standard diagnostic procedure for your doctor to order a viral culture when genital herpes is suspected. As noted above, if you have a genital lesion, and your doctor does not perform a viral culture, you should request one. The technique is similar to that you may have seen demonstrated in your high school biology class, when bacteria are grown (cultured) on a nutrient medium in a petri dish.

To perform a viral culture, the doctor will use a sterile swab to retrieve a fluid sample from a lesion. The sample is sent to a laboratory where it is grown for several days in a culture of healthy human cells. If the sample contains HSV, the virus will infect the cells of the culture, causing cellular changes that can be seen with a microscope. Viral culture earned its status as the gold standard for two reasons. It has good sensitivity, which means it works when even small quantities of virus are retrieved by the swab, and it has good specificity, which means it rarely mistakes another virus for HSV. Actually, the specificity of viral culture is so good it can determine if the infection is caused by HSV-1 or HSV-2. Accurate as it may be, however, viral culture is not infallible. The culture sample must be carefully handled and preserved. Even if herpes lesions are present, the period of viral shedding may be over, in which case the culture will come back negative. We call this a "false negative"— the test says no HSV; nonetheless, the patient has genital herpes. *From 20 to 50 percent of negative HSV cultures may be false negatives.*

It also takes anywhere from two to seven days to get viral culture results back from the laboratory. So, while viral culture can provide almost certain confirmation of genital herpes, and tell us which HSV serotype is responsible, it really isn't all that useful at the practical level of treatment. If genital herpes is suspected, your doctor will probably start drug therapy right away and use the results of the viral culture to guide future treatment decisions. If, for example, the culture reveals you have genital herpes caused by HSV-1, you and your doctor will know that your infection is less likely to recur than if it were caused by HSV-2. This may contribute to your peace of mind and influence your decisions about long-term therapy (see Section 3.4, Managing recurrent infection). You'll also have the consolation of knowing that the risk of asymptomatic shedding (presence of virus without lesions) is greatly reduced if you have HSV-1 in the genital area rather than HSV-2.

Antigen-Detection Tests. An often-used alternative to culture is antigen detection. Unlike the culture method, this test doesn't require growing the virus but rather seeks to identify HSV by way of a reliable marker— the presence of antigens, fragments of the virus that are known to stimulate the immune response. These tests rival the culture for sensitivity and specificity, they can be done more quickly, and are sometimes cheaper. The potential downside is that they don't provide a way to determine whether the sample represents infection with HSV-1 or HSV-2.

Direct fluorescence antibody testing. Direct fluorescence antibody (FA) testing is faster than viral culture, but it still requires that a swab-sample be sent to a laboratory. FA testing detects the proteins of HSV. It is quicker than viral culture but slightly less sensitive.

Tzanck test. A Tzanck test involves the scraping of cells from lesions, staining them with a dye, and examining them under a microscope. To the trained eye, cellular changes characteristic of HSV infection may be apparent. The Tzanck can be completed relatively quickly, but it is subjective and best reserved for experienced specialists such as dermatologists and pathologists. Also, it cannot distinguish HSV-1 and HSV-2, nor can it distinguish either HSV serotype from VZV (varicella zoster virus), the herpesvirus that causes chickenpox and shingles. This test, therefore, is not particularly useful.

Polymerase chain reaction. The most sensitive test for confirming the presence of HSV at a particular anatomic site is polymerase chain reaction (PCR). Unfortunately PCR technology is not widely available; its principal use so far has been for research into the epidemiology of HSV infection. There are presently no recommendations for its use in the diagnosis of genital herpes, but it will probably become a part of the standard diagnostic arsenal in time.

Serologic testing. All the tests mentioned above are used to detect virus or viral antigens at the site of infection, and in the past culture and antigen tests have been viewed as the preferred tests during an initial attack of herpes. Serologic tests, by contrast, detect antibodies in the blood, and it can take from a few weeks to months for these antibodies to develop. If a person goes from being HSV seronegative to HSV seropositive in association with symptoms, the infection is a primary episode. That's one use for serologic tests. Beyond this, however, serologic assays can be very effective in discovering HSV infections that are already established, and the latest tests may be useful as an aid in diagnosing first episodes as well.

Serologic testing for herpes is a confusing issue. The tests used by many laboratories do not distinguish between HSV-1 and HSV-2; they react with either virus. This poses a problem if you've ever had an HSV-1 infection: the test cannot detect a new HSV-2 infection. Within the last ten years, however, researchers have perfected a number of tests that can distinguish between HSV-1 and HSV-2. That's what we mean by "type-specific." The "gold standard" is known as the **Western blot,** developed by scientists at the University of Washington.

An important diagnostic advance, this assay is very useful in determining if you acquired HSV-2 recently or in the past. It can tell us if you have antibodies to HSV-1 only, HSV-2 only, or both serotypes.

A number of biotechnology companies are in the process of developing and bringing to market serologic tests that have similar capabilities but can be done more quickly and cheaply. One of these newer assays, in fact, the POCkit™ HSV-2 Rapid Test (Diagnology) offers the convenience of a blot test that can be done in the doctor's office with a fingerprick and a collection kit, with results in ten minutes. The test looks specifically for HSV-2 antibodies. It's already available in Europe and recently received approval in the United States. According to some experts, this test is actually better at detecting recent herpes infections than some of the more expensive assays.

However quickly the technology moves, the bottom line is that accurate type-specific serologic assays are available and are probably worth mentioning to your health care provider. You can get more information on how to obtain these tests in Appendix B.

2.74 The Importance of Testing for Other STDs

Testing for herpes is essential to confirm the diagnosis of genital herpes. In some situations, tests for other STDs may also be ordered. Sexually transmitted diseases, by definition, are acquired and passed on through sexual activity. If you've acquired genital herpes, there's an increased risk you may also have contracted syphilis, gonorrhea, chlamydia, or another STD. It's also a good idea to go ahead and have an HIV/AIDS test. HIV/AIDS is, after all, a sexually transmitted disease. Herpes simplex viruses and other infectious agents that cause STDs don't care who they strike. Never allow yourself to believe "Oh, it couldn't happen to me." As statistics show, it happens to a great many of us every year.

2.8 COMPLICATIONS

Genital herpes, despite the extreme physical discomfort it produces in some patients, is usually self-limiting (meaning it will resolve on its own) and only rarely causes serious short- or long-term complications. Complications, when they do occur, tend to be associated with primary

TABLE 2.8 COMPLICATIONS OF GENITAL HERPES:
A PARTIAL LIST

Complication	Description
Psychosocial morbidity	Negative emotional and psychological effects of being diagnosed and living with genital herpes. Among the most common complications of genital herpes. Can be serious and long-lasting. See section 3.1, "How Did You Feel When You Got the News?"
Superinfection (fungal/ bacterial)	Occurs when herpes lesions become infected with fungus or bacteria, much as a cut or any other wound might become infected. Also, about 10% of women with primary genital herpes develop vaginal candidiasis (yeast) at the same time, a complication even more common among diabetic women with primary genital herpes.
Extragenital lesions	Herpetic lesions on nongenital surfaces: legs, buttocks, perianal region. Seen in about 20% of primary first episodes. Extragenital lesions can recur and are an underrecognized source of transmission.
Necrotic cervicitis	Almost all women with primary genital herpes also have herpetic infection of the cervix. It can become severe, progressing to a condition called necrotic cervicitis. The symptoms include vaginal discharge; difficult urination; pelvic, genital, or abdominal pain; and constitutional symptoms (fever, headache, malaise, muscle aches, loss of appetite). Healing is spontaneous and usually complete in 2–3 weeks.
Herpetic urethritis	Affects 30–40% of men and more than 80% of women with primary genital herpes. Causes pain during urination.
Herpetic whitlow	Painful HSV infection of the fingertip that can recur. See Appendix A.

Complication	Description
HSV tonsillitis/ pharyngitis	Sore throat, concurrent with primary HSV-1 or HSV-2 genital herpes. Occurs in 10–30% of patients. Constitutional symptoms and swollen lymph nodes in the neck are common. See Appendix A.
Keratoconjunctivitis	HSV infection of the eye. An important complication. See Appendix A.
Anorectal herpes	HSV infection of the perianal region and rectum. Seen with increasing frequency. Symptoms include severe local pain and pain in the anal canal. HSV infection can occur deeper in the rectum and cause HSV proctitis. May arise as a complication of primary genital herpes, but most cases are the result of anal intercourse. More often seen in homosexual men. High likelihood of recurrence.
Meningitis	HSV infection of the meninges (the membranes that cover the brain and spinal cord, causing headache and other symptoms). See Appendix A.

episodes of infection. Table 2.8 briefly outlines some of these complications; several are discussed in greater detail in Appendix A, "Nongenital HSV Infections."

2.9 NEONATAL HERPES (HSV INFECTION IN THE NEWBORN)

2.91 Incidence and Acquisition

The most medically traumatic aspect of genital herpes is transmission of the virus to the newborn, **neonatal herpes.** Unlike the majority of HSV infections, neonatal herpes is always a crisis: more than 50 percent of HSV-infected newborns die or are likely to have serious and long-lasting neurological complications. Fortunately, the annual incidence of neonatal herpes is quite low. Estimates of the overall incidence of neonatal herpes range from 1 in 2,000 to 1 in 5,000 deliveries, although in some areas of the country it may be as high as 1 in 1,500 or as low as 1 in 20,000. The local incidence of neonatal HSV infection depends on the local prevalence of genital herpes.

Recent studies indicate that the risk of neonatal transmission from women with a history of genital HSV infection is *very, very low*. This is especially true if the health care provider knows the mother has herpes. It's one reason why diagnosis of HSV infection is so important.

The HSV **serostatus** of the mother (i.e., whether she has antibodies to the herpes virus) is the most important risk factor for neonatal herpes. Women with long-standing genital HSV infection only infrequently transmit the virus to their babies because these women have developed a full immune response to HSV and actually transmit antibodies to the baby in the womb. This appears to give the newborn protection against HSV present in the birth canal at the time of delivery. Even if the baby is exposed to HSV during birth, antibodies acquired from its mother can protect against infection.

By contrast, women who acquire herpes *during pregnancy* often do not have time to develop a full immune response and transfer protection to the child in the womb. Thus, the highest risk of neonatal transmission occurs in women who experience a primary herpes infection during pregnancy. The baby exposed to HSV at birth without any protective antibodies on board is much more vulnerable to infection. For this reason, a woman who is seronegative for HSV but whose partner is positive is well advised to take extra care to avoid infection during pregnancy, especially during the third trimester. Though statistically less significant, there are also risks associated with primary episodes during the first trimester. Severe primaries carry the risk that virus may be spread to the baby through the placenta. This condition is so rare, however, that testing such as amniocentesis is not useful.

Admittedly, many couples do not know the HSV serostatus of one or both partners. That's why a number of opinion leaders in the field are raising the question of serologic testing to screen all pregnant women and their partners.

For the time being, the standard approach to managing herpes in a pregnant woman includes notifying the midwife or obstetric professional about the patient's history of herpes. A normal vaginal delivery is anticipated, but it's a good idea to discuss what may need to be done in the event the mother-to-be has a herpes outbreak at the same time labor begins. In such a case, the standard of care is to perform a cesarean section delivery to prevent the baby from coming into contact with significant quantities of virus. Another issue is the use of fetal scalp monitors. There is some evidence to suggest that the use of this type of monitor increases the risk of HSV transmission to the newborn. Thus, fetal scalp monitors should be used only when absolutely necessary.

Are outbreaks during pregnancy a problem? Up to 84 percent of women with a history of recurrent genital herpes will have at least one recurrence during pregnancy. This, in and of itself, is not a matter of great concern. The critical issue is *timing*, not frequency. Many women are under the mistaken impression that because they have genital herpes, they must undergo cesarean section. Not true. Only for women experiencing a *symptomatic episode* of genital herpes near the time of delivery — whether it is a primary, nonprimary, or recurrent episode — does standard procedure call for delivering the baby by cesarean section. This is done within four hours of the mother's water breaking. In the womb, the baby is protected from infection to some extent by the membranous amniotic sac. When this sac ruptures around the time of delivery (i.e., when the mother's water breaks) the baby is more easily exposed to virus from the cervix.

For women with a history of recurrent genital herpes but no symptoms at the time of delivery and no other complications that would require cesarean section, a normal vaginal delivery is recommended.

part

THREE

CYNTHIA'S STORY

Part Three

~

Cynthia waited until dinner was over and the dishes had been cleared. Then she invited Brian to join her in the living room. "I have something I need to talk over with you," she said.

When they were comfortably seated, at opposite ends of the couch, she began. "I want you to promise you'll let me finish what I have to say before you start asking questions, okay?"

Brian shrugged and made a face like *"Well, what else would I do?"*

"Promise," Cynthia said.

"I promise."

"Alright, you know I went to see a doctor this morning to see about that yeast infection I've had for the past few days," Cynthia said tentatively, picking at a loose thread on the arm of the couch with her fingernail. "Well, it's not a yeast infection. It never was. I lied to you." Cynthia told him about the Thursday night two weeks earlier when she had first experienced the discomfort in her vaginal area and how rapidly it had intensified, eventually becoming so severe that she couldn't sleep. At first, she said, she thought it was just another yeast infection, particularly in light of their sexual activity over Labor Day weekend.

Brian sat quietly as she described her other symptoms and the anxiety that came over her when she began to realize this was no mere yeast infection, but he wasn't entirely comfortable.

"So I went to see my gynecologist, first thing, the next morning," she said. "And there's just no easy way to tell you this, but Dr. Charles says I have genital herpes. And I went to see another doctor today at the Midtown Women's Clinic, and he agreed. But Brian, I want you to understand and believe me —*I have never, ever been unfaithful to you. I have never, ever cheated on you.*

"Actually," she continued, after a second's pause. "Dr. Foster, the doctor I saw today, is pretty certain I caught it from you." She expected Brian to say something, but he remained silent.

"Please understand!" she said. "I'm not accusing you of anything. Dr. Foster says you could've had it for years and not known. It's like you're a carrier, but you don't get any physical effects from it. But you could, later. It could change, and you could start having physical outbreaks, just like that. They don't know why it changes."

Brian had remained perfectly still and expressionless as Cynthia concluded her story. "It's a sexually transmitted disease, Brian," she said softly. "I haven't had sex with anyone but you for four years."

After a few moments silence, Cynthia spoke again, softly, "Well . . . say something."

"Oh. Is it my turn now? Do I get to talk now? Well, first I want you to promise you'll let me finish what I . . ."

Cynthia waved her right hand and shook her head to cut him off. "Don't," she said, seriously. "That's not funny." She sniffled slightly, and intercepted a tear at the corner of her eye with the edge of her right palm. "I'm trying to do the right thing here. It's as much your problem as it is mine. You've got it too, and you should talk to a doctor. Dr. Foster says you can get a special blood test to confirm it."

In a calm, even tone, Brian answered, "I don't need any *test*. I don't have herpes. If I had it, I'd know. And just for the record, I'd like to state that I have *never, ever* been unfaithful to you in the four years we've been together."

"I'm not accusing you of anything!"

"I know you're not accusing me," Brian continued, "but you did raise the issue. So I want that on the table, up front, okay?"

Cynthia nodded and wiped her eye again. "You're wrong, though.

You've probably had it for years and not known it, and really, it's a wonder I didn't catch it before now."

Brian just shook his head. "Cindy, look at the evidence here. How many people in this room have been diagnosed with herpes?"

She thought he was just being rhetorical, but after a couple of seconds, it became obvious that he actually expected her to respond, so with as sarcastic a look as she could muster, she slowly raised her hand into the air.

"Honey," he said, "all I'm trying to do is get you to take an objective look at the evidence. If anyone in this room has had herpes for years without knowing, it's you."

She shook her head emphatically. "No! You're wrong. Both Dr. Foster and Dr. Charles say I have a primary infection. That means you gave it to me. And if you get a type-specific blood test, you'll see. Talk to Dr. Foster. He'll tell you. If you get a blood test . . ."

"Cynthia, didn't you just say a person can have it for years and not have any physical signs of infection?" Brian asked calmly.

"Yes."

"Then how can you say, beyond a shadow of a doubt, that you haven't been infected for years, since before we met." He paused and continued, "I trust you. I don't suspect for a minute that you've ever cheated on me. I just think you have to look at the facts. What do they say on 'ER'? 'If you hear hoof beats, look for horses, not zebras.'"

～

Cynthia tried to explain the difference between a primary infection and a recurrence but quickly realized she couldn't remember all of what Dr. Foster had told her, only that primary infections tend to be more severe. "If you really want to know the truth, Brian," she said in resignation, "you can have a blood test done."

"And what would that prove?" he asked.

"If you have antibodies to the genital herpes virus, it would prove that what I've been saying is true."

"Not if you've had the virus all along it wouldn't," Brian said, raising his voice slightly. "If I have herpes, it's because I got it from you. I could have gotten it from you any time over the last four years and never known it—you said so yourself—a person can have it for years and never know. If I got it from you, wouldn't I have those antibodies too? Or suppose we've *both* had it for years, since before we met. Isn't that a possibility? And yours suddenly decides to flare up, and it doesn't have anything to do with me? I'm sorry, but I don't see that the presence of antibodies..."

"ALRIGHT!" Cynthia yelled back angrily, covering her ears with her hands. "Alright. Forget it. I have herpes. You don't. Period. End." She pulled her bare feet up onto the couch and wrapped her arms tightly around her legs.

Brian's tone was instantly conciliatory, "Cindy, let's not fight about this. It doesn't matter anyway. I don't care if you have herpes. It doesn't change anything between us.

"Come on," he said, reaching out to her, but she refused to look at him or acknowledge the gesture. "Come on. Forget it. I still love you as much as I ever did. Okay, you lied about the yeast infection this past weekend, but that was for my protection—I appreciate that. You told me the truth tonight, and I know it was a really tough thing to do. That was very brave. I mean it. But let's just drop it, okay? It's no big deal."

"Easy for you to say," Cynthia mumbled. "You don't know what it's like."

∼

Later that night, when she had calmed down and they had just climbed into bed, she tried to bring up the subject of the vaccine study. She figured Brian wouldn't qualify but thought it might be a way to get him tested and prove to him that he was infected.

"Forget it," he said. "I have no intention of becoming a pharmaceutical guinea pig."

"You're not concerned about catching herpes?"

"Sure I'm concerned."

"But you won't take advantage of this new vaccine. I don't get it. Did you understand what I told you about condoms? They may not do any good. No one knows for sure. Are you willing to take that chance every time we have sex?"

"Cynthia," Brian said wearily, "I don't want to talk about this anymore. I'm tired, and I've got a very important meeting tomorrow morning at nine o'clock. So for the sake of my career and our future financial security, will you, for the love of God, *please,* give it rest." He raised himself up on one elbow and looked her in the eye. "In sickness and in health — that's the deal, right? Understand. I'm sorry you have herpes. I'm sorry you suffered so badly when I was in San Diego. You should've told me then, over the phone. At least I could have tried to comfort you. But the truth is, I don't really care if you have herpes, not for my sake. It doesn't matter to me. It doesn't change the way I feel about you. If I get it, I get it. I'll deal with it. We can talk about the condom thing later. But I am not, under any circumstances, going to expose myself to some experimental vaccine, and I'm not interested in talking to your Dr. Foster, okay? Stop obsessing over this. It's not that big a deal."

⁓

Cynthia's Friday follow-up visit with Dr. Charles was less than she'd hoped for. The blood sample, it turned out, had been for a syphilis test, not a Western blot serology. "We just wanted to make sure whoever gave you herpes didn't give you a little something extra at the same time. But you're fine."

Cynthia told Dr. Charles about her consultation with Dr. Foster, and just as Dr. Foster had predicted, Dr. Charles was not in the least offended when Cynthia said she was going to switch over to the Midtown Clinic for future gynecological care. She promised to come back, however, if and when she became pregnant. He wished her the best, and they parted amicably.

⁓

In late November, Cynthia experienced her first recurrence of genital herpes. She felt it coming a day in advance and was able to initiate therapy before the lesions appeared. Her symptoms were much milder than before — mainly vulvar pain and moderate urinary difficulties. She phoned the Clinic and got an immediate appointment with Dr. Foster. His examination was thorough. He cultured her lesions, and when he learned she hadn't yet had a type-specific serologic test, he ordered a Western blot.

Later, sitting in his office, they reviewed her treatment options for the management of recurrent infection, and he suggested she hold off on suppressive therapy until they could establish how often her outbreaks would occur.

Dr. Foster had noticed that Cynthia seemed a little distracted or depressed. Recalling their first conversation he decided to ask how things had gone when she told Brian about her infection. She rolled her eyes.

"He wouldn't listen. He said he didn't have herpes, and that was that. I told him all the stuff you told me about dormant virus and asymptomatic shedding, but he wouldn't listen. I told him he should have a blood test. He said no. I even tried to trick him into it by getting him interested in the vaccine study, but he wouldn't discuss it. He said he was not interested in becoming a drug-company guinea pig. End of story. I decided to just let it go, y'know? Enough is enough. Plus, he's really been kinda great through this whole business. Very little has changed. Basically, he says it doesn't matter to him that I have herpes. He still loves me as much as ever and says he doesn't care if he gets infected — that he'll deal with it if and when the time comes. Of course, you and I know that's not going to happen. He's already got it, sure as the world."

Dr. Foster nodded, "I strongly suspect he does. It would take a type-specific blood test to confirm it, but I gather that's out of the question."

"Definitely," Cynthia agreed emphatically. "I guess I should feel lucky. At least he knows about it. We still have sex. Not as often as before, but that's more me than him. Sometimes when I think of sex now, I start thinking about herpes, and I remember the pain of that first episode, and it just turns me off, completely. But I know how lucky I am. I've got Brian, and he accepts me as I am. I just can't imagine telling anyone else about this. I can't imagine finding anyone else who would want me now. And I don't want to be alone."

"Well, you were lucky. You had a solid relationship before all this happened. I've known women who caught herpes in the early days of a sexual relationship and actually wound up marrying the man who infected them, men they barely knew and, in some cases, didn't even like all that much, *solely* because they were afraid no one else would have them. It's heartbreaking to see that because I know from professional experience that the process of emotional adjustment takes time. You have to give yourself time."

Cynthia managed a weak smile. "Those women feel trapped," she said. "That is sad."

"So how is Brian adapting to condoms," Dr. Foster asked. "I know last time you said he really hates to wear them."

"He isn't . . . doesn't. He said he'd rather risk catching herpes than go back to using condoms. So now I guess every time we have sex, he must feel like he's playing Russian roulette. I keep thinking, *'Have the damned blood test, fool'* but I don't want to push him on that subject any more. Things aren't perfect, by any means, but I don't want to rock the boat." Then she added, with a weak smile, "I guess I'm not so different from those other women you were talking about. I don't want to be alone either."

chapter three

GENITAL HERPES: TREATMENT, MANAGEMENT, AND PREVENTION

$\sim$

3.1 HOW DID YOU FEEL WHEN YOU FIRST GOT THE NEWS?

A diagnosis of genital herpes can be emotionally devastating. Anger, guilt, shame, fear, frustration, isolation, and depression are not uncommon reactions. There's no quick fix, but it's crucial that you try to work past these negative feelings. Generally, people have their most intense emotional response during the initial episode, sometimes because of the physical aspects and sometimes because of the social and emotional impact. Newly diagnosed patients may start to feel better after the symptoms subside and may even yield to wishful thinking—*maybe their infection will not recur.* But with the first symptomatic recurrence, the reality of life with genital herpes reasserts itself, and old psychic wounds may reopen.

In 1993, the American Social Health Association (ASHA), a private nonprofit agency dedicated to the prevention and control of STDs, published a survey of patient attitudes about genital herpes. Almost 3,000 people with genital herpes answered questions about their feelings, both during the initial episode and in the 12 months prior to the survey. The majority had had herpes for more than six years.

Depression, fear of rejection, feelings of isolation, fear of discovery, and self-destructive feelings were common during the initial episode, and those feelings persisted, although to a lesser degree, into the year preceding the survey. Although the participants were not randomly selected and the results may not be typical of the average herpes patient, the ASHA study serves as a poignant reminder that herpes still carries a social stigma and requires a period of adjustment for many patients — even in the 1990s. The important things to note here are the range of feelings reported and the fact that the intensity of those feelings lessened with time. Results are summarized in Figure 3.1.

Perhaps the biggest concern of people with herpes is the fear of transmitting the infection to a current or future sexual partner. This fear reflects the natural desire not to inflict injury on another person as well as apprehension over the impact of transmission on a relationship. As our ongoing story of Cynthia and Brian shows, the sudden and unexpected appearance of herpes in a relationship can be traumatic and disruptive. Fortunately, we have learned a good deal over the past two decades about reducing the risk of transmission.

Honesty and openness in the early stages of a relationship can help allay the fear of transmission. Communication is the key, but be advised, many people have difficulty discussing sexual issues, and some of the most likely questions may not be readily answerable: *Where, when, and from whom did you contract herpes? How many recurrences will you have? When will they happen?*

Maybe you don't need any help dealing with these questions, but don't lie to yourself. If you are having trouble adjusting, talk to your health care provider. He or she may be able to offer the level of counseling you need or can certainly refer you to an appropriate, reliable alternative source. In many metropolitan areas, support groups have been organized to give people with herpes a place to go and talk to other people with herpes. Chapter 5 of this book also lists a number of resources for additional information and assistance with the emotional adjustment.

Don't panic. Don't yield to desperation. Genital herpes doesn't have to mean the end of your social life. People with herpes flirt, date, have

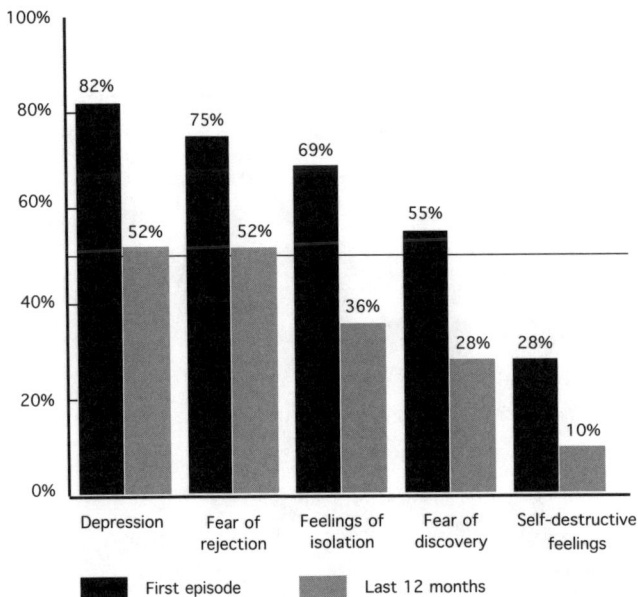

FIGURE 3.1 Feelings during HSV episodes. (From Catotti, 1993)

sex, fall in love, get married, and raise children, just like people who don't have herpes (and just like people who have herpes but *don't know* they have it).

3.2 ANTIVIRAL THERAPY: WHAT IT CAN AND CAN'T DO

You'll hear it said, time and again, that genital herpes is incurable. Though technically accurate, "incurable" is an unfortunate choice of words. It implies a continuous disease-state of endless suffering, and that's just not typical of genital herpes, especially if you understand how to manage your infection. True, once you have an HSV infection, it's with you for life, but that's also true of herpes zoster (the cause of chickenpox) and Epstein-Barr virus (the cause of mononucleosis), and neither chickenpox nor mono are diseases most people think of as incurable. The only difference is, HSV-1 and HSV-2 are a great deal more likely to reactivate and cause recurrent infection.

Antiviral therapy for an initial episode of genital herpes (primary or nonprimary) can shorten the duration of many symptoms, shorten the duration of viral shedding (the time when you are most contagious), and speed the healing of lesions. It would be great if antiviral therapy were also able to prevent HSV from permanently setting up shop in the nerve ganglia, but none of the currently available drugs can accomplish this. One drug, famciclovir, has been shown to prevent the establishment of latency in laboratory animals, but it remains to be seen whether that result will be repeated in humans.

Even though antiviral treatment *during* a first episode has no effect on the subsequent frequency or severity of recurrent infections, antiviral therapy can be used after the virus has established latency to reduce the frequency and severity of recurrences and prevent them altogether in many cases. Antiviral therapy will probably also be shown to reduce the risk of transmission to others by reducing the frequency of asymptomatic viral shedding (when active virus is present on genital surfaces but you don't know because you have no symptoms).

How you use antiviral therapy to manage an established infection will be for you to decide—once you understand the strategic options.

3.3 TREATING THE FIRST SYMPTOMATIC EPISODE

Your first symptomatic episode of genital herpes may be the result of very recent exposure to HSV, or it may simply be the first symptomatic recurrence of a latent infection you never knew you had. In either case, the standard course of treatment is the same.

After taking your medical history and conducting a thorough examination, if your doctor suspects you have genital herpes, he or she will probably begin antiviral drug therapy right away, without waiting for test results from the laboratory. The sooner treatment is started, the more effective it's likely to be. Even if test results come back negative, your doctor may advise you to continue therapy. A false-negative result (the failure to detect HSV) is always a possibility, and diagnosis is a multifaceted process. Usually, time will tell if the diagnosis is accurate; symptomatic first episodes tend to be followed by recurrent outbreaks, often within a couple of months.

According to the U.S. Centers for Disease Control and Prevention, three highly effective antiviral drugs are currently available to treat first episodes of genital herpes: **acyclovir** (brand name: Zovirax®); **valacyclovir** (brand name: Valtrex®); and **famciclovir** (brand name: Famvir®). Patent protection on acyclovir expired in April 1997, and generic versions are now available. While all three of these medications are effective and safe, and all three are viable treatment options, it may be useful to know a little about how they were developed and how they work.

Acyclovir was the first antiviral drug to be developed and marketed for genital herpes. It does not kill HSV; rather, it stops the virus from reproducing. Acyclovir was a great leap forward for people with herpes because it finally gave medical professionals a way to alleviate symptoms and gain a measure of control over the infection. Acyclovir was initially used to shorten first episodes and to help shorten severe recurrences. The next major milestone in herpes therapy came with the discovery that a daily dose of acyclovir can actually suppress reactivation altogether in many patients. Even people who were having up to 12 outbreaks per year could take a daily dose of acyclovir and achieve an 80 percent decrease in recurrences. Subsequently, we learned that up to 20 percent of patients on daily acyclovir had no outbreaks at all.

One of the drawbacks to acyclovir was that only 15 to 20 percent of the drug was actually absorbed by the body. So researchers went to work developing similar compounds that would be better absorbed and might offer some therapeutic advantages over acyclovir, such as longer-lasting impact and less frequent dosing. These efforts produced two relatively new drugs: valacyclovir and famciclovir.

Valacyclovir is the prodrug of acyclovir. It is converted to acyclovir in the body. As a result, more acyclovir is absorbed by the body and delivered to the sites of infection. This strategy of boosting absorption by administering a prodrug has also been employed in the development of **famciclovir,** whose active ingredient is a compound called penciclovir.

All three drugs — acyclovir, valacyclovir, and famciclovir — are now approved to treat a variety of HSV infections. The U.S. Centers for Disease Control's recommended antiviral regimens for first episodes of genital herpes are given in Table 3.3.

In our clinical experience, both valacyclovir and famciclovir offer therapeutic advantages over acyclovir. If you think you would have difficulty adhering to a regimen that required a mid-day dose, valacyclovir (on a morning/evening schedule) might be a better choice for you.

All three currently available antivirals have excellent safety profiles. As observed in placebo-controlled trials, the most common adverse events reported with these drugs included the following: nausea, vomiting, headache, diarrhea, indigestion, fatigue, stomach ache, loss of energy, and loss of appetite. The rates at which these events were reported were very low. (**Placebo-controlled** means one group of patients receives active drug, and another group receives an inactive "sugar pill," or placebo.)

Note on adverse events and side effects: "Adverse event" and "side effect" are not synonymous terms. "Adverse event" refers to any negative physical or psychological experience a patient reports while taking a drug. If that event can be proved to be caused by the drug, it can then be called a side effect. In other words, all side effects are adverse events, but not all adverse events are side effects. In clinical studies, every adverse event a patient reports while taking the experimental drug is

TABLE 3.3 RECOMMENDED ORAL ANTIVIRAL REGIMENS FOR FIRST EPISODES OF GENITAL HERPES

Name	Brand	Regimen*
Acyclovir	Zovirax®	400 mg, 3 times daily (every 8 hours) for 7–10 days*
Acyclovir	Zovirax®	200 mg, 5 times daily (at 4-hour intervals—8 a.m., noon, 4 p.m., 8 p.m., and midnight) for 7–10 days*
Famciclovir	Famvir®	250 mg, 3 times daily (every 8 hours) for 7–10 days*
Valacyclovir	Valtrex®	1000 mg, 2 times daily (every 12 hours) for 7–10 days*

*Therapy should be continued for 7–10 days or until all lesions have healed.

listed, regardless of whether the event was actually caused by the drug. This is to make certain that no real side effects go unnoticed. The adverse events listed above for acyclovir, valacyclovir, and famciclovir are those that were reported the most often in placebo-controlled clinical studies. But the fact that these events are listed doesn't necessarily mean you should expect to experience them or even that they can be positively associated with the drug — only that they are possibilities.

3.4 MANAGING RECURRENT INFECTION

As painful and unpleasant as the first episode of genital herpes may be, it can only happen once. Eventually, with or without antiviral therapy, symptoms subside, and lesions disappear. This begins a period of high anxiety for many patients as they wonder, *Will it come back and, if so, when? How often? How bad will it be?* These are questions no one can answer in advance. The simple statistical realities are these:

- If you have a symptomatic first episode of genital herpes due to HSV-2, in the 12 months that follow you have about a 90 percent chance of at least one recurrence; about a 40 percent chance of 6 or more recurrences; and about a 20 percent chance of 10 or more recurrences. Overall the average recurrence rate is about four episodes per year. *Note: These estimates were derived from patients receiving no antiviral therapy to suppress recurrent infection.*
- HSV-1 is less likely to recur than HSV-2. The average recurrence rate for genital herpes due to HSV-1 is about one episode per year.

If you've had a symptomatic first episode of genital herpes, the odds are it was caused by HSV-2, and the odds are you *will* have recurrent outbreaks. The real question is, what can you do about it?

First, you need to learn about *your* infection and its pattern of recurrence. Many doctors encourage their patients to keep a herpes diary in the first year, to document recurrences and to track prodromal symptoms (early symptoms that occur in advance of each outbreak). Learning to recognize your own prodrome is an important skill that will aid you in the management of your disease. The prodrome is a very individualized phenomenon. Yours will be unique, and you will learn to recognize it from experience. (Typical prodromal symptoms are described in Section 2.54.)

A herpes diary is also a convenient place to jot down questions you want to ask your doctor at the next visit. If you're like most people, the diagnosis came as a shock, and you really didn't pay close attention to everything that was said after you heard, "You have genital herpes." This reaction is so common that doctors generally are advised to schedule a follow-up visit within a week or two of the initial diagnosis, in order to review instructions to the patient and to answer any questions that may have occurred to the patient after the news has had time to sink in.

If you keep an accurate diary, you will be better able to gain a sense of your infection: how often it recurs, how you feel in the 24–48 hours before a recurrence, and what situations and stimuli seem to "trigger" an outbreak. Reactivation of latent HSV can be triggered by any of the following: fever, menstruation, emotional stress, nutritional stress, lack of sleep, sexual intercourse (particularly "rigorous" or poorly lubricated intercourse), ultraviolet light (mainly sunlight), and trauma to the sacral ganglia (from surgery or a back injury).

Your doctor could treat each recurrent episode the same way he or she treated your initial episode — you return to the doctor each time you have symptoms; the doctor says, "Yes, it's herpes again" and writes you a prescription. But this is an inefficient, expensive, and medically inferior way to treat recurrences. It leaves you completely dependent on your doctor for medical intervention each time an outbreak occurs, and it delays treatment, which compromises effectiveness.

Think beyond the idea of treatment, which regards each new episode as an isolated medical event and uses antiviral therapy only in reaction to an outbreak. Instead, start thinking in terms of *management,* which allows you to use antiviral therapy more aggressively. Management means control. It means you take responsibility for your own infection, including the possibility of its spread to others.

There are two strategies for the use of antiviral therapy in the management of recurrent genital herpes: **episodic therapy** and **suppressive therapy.** Through the years, you will probably use both strategies, at different times, depending on the circumstances of your personal life and the recurrence patterns of your infection, which can be expected to change over time. Both strategies are described below in Sections 3.41 and 3.42, and a hypothetical case history illustrating their integration over a 12-year period in one patient's life is outlined in Section 3.43.

Each patient's response is unique, but if properly used, antiviral therapy may achieve the following:

Episodic therapy (taking antiviral medication only when an outbreak threatens or is ongoing)
- may stop some recurrent outbreaks in the early stages
- may reduce the severity of outbreaks and speed the healing of lesions

Suppressive therapy (taking antiviral medication every day, even in the absence of symptoms)
- may reduce the frequency of recurrences, completely eliminating them for some patients for extended periods
- may reduce the frequency of asymptomatic shedding
- probably will reduce the risk of transmitting the virus to your partner(s) through the combined effect of the above

3.41 Episodic Antiviral Therapy for Recurrent Genital Herpes

Successful episodic therapy depends, to a great extent, on your ability to predict a recurrence of genital herpes by the onset of prodromal symptoms. Episodic therapy should be initiated at the first prodromal sign or symptom of recurrent infection. The prodrome may precede overt symptomatic infection by only a few hours, so it's best to have a supply of antiviral drug on hand.

It may not always be possible for you to predict a recurrence. This does not represent a failure on your part. Some people never have any identifiable prodromal symptoms. Nonetheless, antiviral therapy is more effective when initiated early. So if you decide to use episodic antiviral therapy to manage recurrent genital herpes, it's best that you have the drug available to you at all times — at home and when you travel.

The U.S. Centers for Disease Control's recommended antiviral regimens for episodic therapy of recurrent genital herpes are given in Table 3.41 below. According to the data reviewed by the FDA, the most common adverse events reported with these drugs were not serious; did not occur frequently, compared with placebo; and were, in many cases, indistinguishable from the symptoms of genital herpes.

As we've explained, the primary role of episodic therapy is to alleviate the symptoms of an outbreak already in progress. What is preferable, of course, is to abort outbreaks completely with episodic therapy. So far, only one drug has been shown to abort episodes when taken at the first symptom of a recurrence. In one clinical trial, episodic therapy with valacyclovir prevented the development of vesicles and ulcerative lesions in 31 percent of patients (Spruance 1996). This is perhaps due to the superior absorption of valacyclovir when compared to acyclovir.

TABLE 3.41 RECOMMENDED ORAL ANTIVIRAL REGIMENS FOR EPISODIC THERAPY OF RECURRENT GENITAL HERPES

Name	Brand	Regimen*
Acyclovir	Zovirax®	200 mg, 5 times daily at 4-hour intervals for 5 days*
Acyclovir	Zovirax®	400 mg, 3 times daily (every 8 hours) for 5 days*
Acyclovir	Zovirax®	800 mg, 2 times daily (every 12 hours) for 5 days*
Famciclovir	Famvir®	125 mg, 2 times daily (every 12 hours) for 5 days*
Valacyclovir	Valtrex®	500 mg, 2 times daily (every 12 hours) for 5 days*

* Episodic therapy should be initiated at the onset of prodromal symptoms (or at the first sign of infection, if no prodrome is detected) and continued for a minimum of 5 days or until all lesions have healed.

3.42 Suppressive Antiviral Therapy for Recurrent Genital Herpes

Suppressive antiviral therapy for recurrent genital herpes (also called prophylactic therapy) involves taking the antiviral drug every day. Patterns of recurrence can change with time, so every 12–24 months patients on suppressive therapy are advised to stop taking the antiviral drug to determine if continued suppressive therapy is needed. Some patients find that even though they continue to need suppressive therapy to control recurrences, they can reduce the dose. Such dosage adjustments should only be undertaken in consultation with your physician. The U.S. Centers for Disease Control's recommended antiviral regimens for suppressive therapy are given in Table 3.42.

PREVENTING, OR REDUCING THE FREQUENCY OF, SYMPTOMATIC RECURRENCES

Suppressive therapy with acyclovir can dramatically reduce the frequency of recurrent genital herpes and in some cases prevent recurrences altogether. This has been shown most convincingly in a study involving 1,146 patients with frequently recurring genital herpes. The patients

TABLE 3.42 RECOMMENDED ORAL ANTIVIRAL REGIMENS FOR SUPPRESSION OF RECURRENT GENITAL HERPES

Name	Brand	Regimen
Acyclovir	Zovirax®	400 mg, 2 times daily (every 12 hours) every day
Famciclovir	Famvir®	250 mg, 2 times daily (every 12 hours) every day
Valacyclovir	Valtrex®	500 mg, once daily (every 24 hours) every day (*Patients with a history of 10 or fewer outbreaks per year*)
Valacyclovir	Valtrex®	1000 mg, once daily (every 24 hours) every day (*Patients with a history of 10 or more outbreaks per year*)

were randomly assigned to one of two treatment groups. Half the patients took acyclovir every day at the recommended dose of two 200 mg capsules every 12 hours; the other half took two capsules every 12 hours that were identical in appearance to acyclovir but contained only an inactive placebo (no drug). Whenever patients in either group experienced a recurrence, they received episodic therapy with acyclovir for 5 days and then returned to the daily regimen to which they were originally assigned. Neither the patients nor their doctors knew who was taking the real drug and who was taking the "sugar pill."

Of the patients taking acyclovir as suppressive therapy, 44 percent had no symptomatic recurrences during the 12-month study, compared with 2 percent of those taking placebo. Among patients taking acyclovir, the average number of symptomatic recurrences fell from about 13 per year to less than 2 per year. In the placebo group the recurrence rate remained close to the prestudy level. See Table 3.421.

All the patients, including those in the placebo group, were given the option of remaining in a long-term study of suppressive therapy with acyclovir; 389 patients completed the 5-year study. Results are shown in Table 3.422.

Reducing the Frequency of Asymptomatic Viral Shedding

Encouraging as it may be to learn that suppressive antiviral therapy can help control or eliminate symptomatic recurrences of genital herpes, a larger problem demands our attention: asymptomatic viral shedding.

Our knowledge of genital herpes has improved considerably over the past two decades. Fifteen to twenty years ago, we believed genital herpes could only be transmitted during symptomatic episodes of infection. We even told people they didn't have to worry about transmitting herpes to their partners between symptomatic recurrences. Today we know that up to 70 percent of new cases of genital herpes are the result of asymptomatic viral shedding, when active virus is present on genital surfaces and neighboring sites but no lesions are visible and no other symptoms are evident. Just five years ago, we thought asymptomatic viral shedding occurred on about 1 out of every 100 days. Today, based on studies using a supersensitive diagnostic technique called polymerase chain

TABLE 3.421 RESULTS OF A PLACEBO-CONTROLLED STUDY OF SUPPRESSIVE ACYCLOVIR IN 1,146 PATIENTS WITH FREQUENT SYMPTOMATIC RECURRENCES OF GENITAL HERPES

	Average number of recurrences at the beginning of the study	Average number of recurrences after 12 months on the study	Patients with no recurrent episodes during the study
Patients taking acyclovir	12.8 per year	1.8 per year	44%
Patients taking placebo	12.7 per year	11.4 per year	2%

(From Mertz 1988)

TABLE 3.422 RESULTS OF A 5-YEAR FOLLOW-UP STUDY OF SUPPRESSIVE ACYCLOVIR FOR RECURRENT SYMPTOMATIC GENITAL HERPES

	AVERAGE NUMBER OF RECURRENCES PER YEAR					
	Prestudy	Year 1	Year 2	Year 3	Year 4	Year 5
210 patients who took acyclovir for all 5 years of the study	12.9	1.7	1.3	1.0	0.9	0.8
179 patients who took placebo in year 1, then acyclovir in years 2–5	12.0	12.5	1.6	1.2	1.0	0.8

(From Goldberg 1993) Includes only those patients who completed the full five years of the study. Note that ex-placebo patients had a dramatic decline in recurrence rate in Year 2 when they started taking acyclovir (from 12.5 per year to 1.6 per year). Also note that the reduction in recurrence rate in both groups was sustained across all years of suppressive therapy.

reaction (or PCR), we believe the frequency of asymptomatic viral shedding may be as high as one out of every five days in some individuals.

If you're like most people with genital herpes, you're concerned about transmitting the infection to others. In one large survey, this concern was expressed by 89 percent of respondents. The fact that 70 percent of transmission results from asymptomatic shedding and the possibility that you may be shedding virus asymptomatically one out of every five days may leave you feeling somewhat helpless. It needn't.

In a recent study (Wald 1996), suppressive antiviral therapy with acyclovir reduced the number of days of asymptomatic viral shedding by 94 percent in women. Theoretically then, daily suppressive acyclovir could reduce the frequency of asymptomatic shedding from about 1 day in 5 to about 1 day in 77. It's logical to assume that reducing the number of days that infectious virus is present on genital surfaces will also reduce the risk of transmission. Although no studies to test this hypothesis have been completed to date, researchers are currently conducting a trial to determine whether valacyclovir can significantly alter the risk of transmission in discordant couples.

3.43 Alternating Use of Episodic and Suppressive Antiviral Therapy

Genital herpes is a lifelong infection. Generally, recurrences become less frequent with time, although it is by no means abnormal for a person's pattern of recurrences to change more than once over the years. Why this happens, we don't know.

If you opt for antiviral therapy, how you use it will largely be a decision for you to make, not your doctor. It depends on the frequency and the severity of your recurrences—but more important, it depends on the circumstances of your personal life. There are no rules in this regard. One person may have four or five recurrences a year that are adequately controlled with episodic therapy, and she may be perfectly satisfied with that strategy. Another person may average three or four recurrences a year but be virtually paralyzed with anxiety over when the next outbreak will occur; he'll probably go with suppressive therapy. One thing to keep in mind when you make your decision, however, is the reduction of asymptomatic shedding with suppressive therapy (and the putative reduction in the risk of transmission)—you lose that benefit if you choose episodic therapy.

The following fictional case study illustrates how a person might integrate both strategies over a period of several years:

Linda contracted genital herpes in 1986, at the age of 23, the summer after graduating from college. Viral culture confirmed that her infection was caused by HSV-2, and the severity of her local and constitutional symptoms strongly suggested that hers was a primary first episode. She was treated with acyclovir, one capsule (200 mg) five times daily, and the initial episode resolved in about two weeks.

In the year that followed, Linda had 12 recurrences, and they were quite painful. At the recommendation of her doctor, she began suppressive therapy with acyclovir in the summer of 1987. For the next 12 months on suppressive therapy, she had no recurrences, so in the summer of 1988, she decided to try switching to episodic therapy. However, her outbreaks resumed their monthly recurrence, just as before, and by Christmas of 1988, she resumed suppressive therapy.

Linda continued suppressive therapy for the next five years, during which time she got married and had two children, although she stopped all antiviral therapy during those times when she was trying to become pregnant and during both pregnancies. Since it also became known in that five-year interval that her husband was infected with HSV-2, the issue of transmission lost its urgency, and in 1993, Linda decided to try episodic therapy once more. Once again, her outbreaks resumed at a rate of about one per month, but they were much less severe than before. By paying close attention to her own prodromal symptoms (and because her recurrences were predictably linked to her period), Linda was able to initiate episodic therapy early. With episodic therapy, her monthly outbreaks were very mild and lasted only a couple of days. After another year she stopped using acyclovir altogether. The monthly outbreaks continued, always in association with her periods, but they weren't painful.

Unfortunately, the marriage didn't last. Linda and her husband divorced in early 1996, and now she is in a relationship with a new partner, Carl. She has told Carl about her infection. He is completely accepting of her but still uneasy about the prospect of contracting genital herpes. Linda's doctor has counseled that merely avoiding intercourse when she is having a symptomatic recurrence is no guarantee Carl will not become infected; they must also consider the risk of transmission from asymptomatic shedding. So even though her outbreaks are now virtually painless, last only a few days, and occur only every three to four months, Linda has decided to resume suppressive therapy out of concern for Carl and their mutual peace of mind. What's more, she has chosen valacyclovir, in the hope that the higher blood levels of acyclovir achieved with valacyclovir will more effectively reduce asymptomatic shedding and further reduce the risk of transmission to her new partner.

3.5 Prevention

Unfortunately, the only 100 percent effective way to prevent the transmission of genital herpes is to abstain from sexual contact altogether. There are, however, a number of less severe steps you can take to reduce the risk, including condoms during intercourse, barrier protection during oral sex, and antiviral therapy to reduce the frequency of asymptomatic viral shedding.

3.51 Single, Sexually Active, No Monogamous Relationship, and No History of Genital Herpes

Any sexually active person not in a monogamous relationship in which the HIV status of both partners has been clinically confirmed should already be practicing safer sex: using condoms for penetrating sex (including fellatio) and kitchen-grade plastic wrap or latex dental dams during cunnilingus.

NOTE ON SPERMICIDES

Many of the health education materials distributed over the last ten years have emphasized the use of spermicides along with condoms for protection against various STDs, including chlamydia, gonorrhea, and AIDS. Spermicides can neutralize bacteria and viruses, and some researchers still advocate their use for STD prevention. However, there is some evidence, such as that found in a recent study by The Population Council, that regular use of spermicides may cause small lesions on mucosal tissue and increase the risk of infection. In all fairness, the jury is still out on this question; nonetheless, our discussion will emphasize other means of risk reduction.

What are the rationales for these measures? Actually, condoms are more effective at stopping the spread of AIDS and certain other STDs than they are against genital herpes, the reason being that HSV-1 and HSV-2 can be shed from or invade areas not covered by a condom.

If you are hoping to go through life without contracting genital herpes, the best thing you can do to reduce your risk, other than practicing safer sex, is keep the number of people with whom you have sex to a minimum. The likelihood of contracting genital herpes increases with your lifetime total of sexual partners. The more people you have sex with, the more likely you are to have sex with a person who has an active HSV-2 infection, and the more likely you are to contract genital herpes.

Maybe you've never experienced any of the symptoms of genital herpes, but you have reason to believe you've been exposed to HSV by a past or current sexual partner. Understanding just how subtle herpes can be, you may be concerned that you have an asymptomatic infection, and you should see an experienced medical professional if symptoms appear. You also have the option of having a type-specific blood test performed, as described in Appendix B.

Remember: An estimated one in four individuals in the United

States over the age of 12 has genital herpes, and the vast majority are unaware of it.

3.52 Single, Sexually Active, No Monogamous Relationship, and Diagnosed with Genital Herpes

Most people who have genital herpes and know they have it want to avoid passing it on to anyone else. If you are a sexually active person with genital herpes who is not in a monogamous relationship, you should already be practicing safer sex to protect yourself from AIDS and other STDs, but there's an additional step you must take to avoid transmitting herpes: **Never have intercourse during a symptomatic episode, not even using a condom.** This prohibition includes the period preceding an outbreak when you first experience prodromal symptoms and lasts until all lesions heal. It's even a good idea to wait an extra couple of days after healing appears complete because the risk of asymptomatic shedding is high immediately after a symptomatic outbreak.

As for the time between recurrences: We used to think genital herpes could only be transmitted during a symptomatic outbreak, but now we know up to 70 percent of cases are caused by asymptomatic viral shedding. The frequency of asymptomatic shedding may be as high as one day out of every five, and even with barrier protection, some risk of transmission remains. This being the case, you face some difficult decisions about telling your prospective partner(s).

Telling a prospective partner you have genital herpes is never easy, but the moral argument for "full disclosure" is rather compelling. Genital herpes is for life, and although usually mild, even when symptomatic, it can be serious under certain circumstances. A person has a right to know he or she is at risk for herpes by having sex with you. And you cannot remove all of the risk by practicing safer sex. You should also be aware that by not telling a prospective partner, you may risk legal action. If your partner contracts genital herpes, and it can be proven that you knew you were infected but didn't warn your partner, you could be sued. The likelihood of a successful legal action of this type is probably slim, but it risks a very public and potentially costly airing of intimate details from your personal life.

How, when, and what to tell a prospective partner is up to you, but it's a discussion that should precede sexual involvement. You'll find a short list of discussion points at the end of Chapter 4.

Choose a quiet, private spot for this conversation, other than the bedroom. You may want to get the ball rolling by raising the issue of sex and sexually transmitted diseases in general. In this era of AIDS, you are well within your rights to inquire about a prospective partner's sexual history. A frank admission of your own genital herpes shows that you are honest and that you care about the other person's well-being. If you didn't care, you wouldn't risk rejection. Expect your prospective partner to be affected by the news, and realize it may take some time for him or her to "process" it. Be prepared to answer questions about prevention and the risk of transmission. You may even consider lending this book to your prospective partner.

The following section (3.53) outlines the steps couples can follow to minimize the risk of transmission in a monogamous relationship.

3.53 Monogamous Relationship, One Partner Has Genital Herpes

Couples concerned about transmission of genital herpes should avoid sexual intercourse and oral sex completely during symptomatic outbreaks, which are known to be times of significant viral shedding. Between outbreaks, there are two major precautions you can take to reduce the risk of transmission. Neither of these precautions is perfect, but each can improve your chances of avoiding transmission. Depending on your level of concern about transmission, your sexual practices, and other personal considerations, you may choose to exercise one or both of these precautions:

1. **Barrier protection.** Use condoms during intercourse and fellatio, and use a cut condom, latex dental dam, or kitchen-grade plastic wrap as a barrier between mouth and genitals during cunnilingus. Condoms are generally effective against STDs and are considered useful (but not perfect) protection against transmission of (and infection by) HSV. However,

viral shedding and infection can occur at sites not covered by a condom, and studies have confirmed that herpes can be transmitted in couples who do use condoms.

2. **Suppressive antiviral therapy**. Most experts believe ongoing studies will show suppressive antiviral therapy reduces the risk of transmission. Full results from these studies should be known in the year 2000.

Before making a decision about either of these precautions, you should consider another variable in the prevention equation: your partner's serostatus (whether he or she has antibodies to HSV-1 or HSV-2). Let's think back to the case study we described in section 3.43. When we left Linda, she was in a new relationship and had decided to resume suppressive antiviral therapy to reduce the risk of transmission to Carl, her partner. We do not know Carl's serostatus. If he were tested for HSV antibodies, the results could be used to guide Linda in her decision. For example: If a type-specific test revealed that Carl had been previously infected with HSV-2, prevention would be a nonissue and suppressive therapy would be unnecessary. If the test showed that Carl had been previously infected with HSV-1, prevention would still be an issue, but they would know that he has partial immunity and would not get a primary infection if transmission did occur.

Another important issue for couples concerned about transmission is the risk associated with oral sex. For illustration, let's imagine two more fictitious couples:

1. Lauren and Robert — Lauren has no history of genital herpes, but her boyfriend, Robert, tells her he has had genital herpes for at least five years. Lauren does not want to perform fellatio on Robert because she is afraid she will acquire an HSV infection of the lips or mouth. This is, indeed, a potential risk. The degree of risk is difficult to gauge without knowing whether Lauren has a pre-existing oral HSV infection. A pre-existing HSV infection would confer some, though not complete, protection. Given the difficulty of assessing the risk of genital-to-oral transmission, many

couples elect to use some form of barrier protection during oral sex.

2. Elyssa and Todd — Todd has a long history of cold sores due to HSV-1, and his lover, Elyssa, is worried she will acquire a genital HSV-1 infection from him during cunnilingus if he is shedding virus asymptomatically in his mouth. In reality, he could pass HSV-1 to her either mouth-to-mouth, when kissing, or mouth-to-genitals, during oral sex. If Elyssa is already infected with HSV-1, however, the risk is minimal. A type-specific serologic test could confirm prior infection with HSV-1.

For information on how to obtain a type-specific serologic test for HSV-1 and HSV-2, see Appendix B, beginning on page 153.

3.54 Pregnant, No History of Genital Herpes

Between 75 and 80 percent of HSV infections of the newborn occur during childbirth; about 5 percent of infections occur in the womb; and the remaining 15 to 20 percent are acquired in the weeks immediately after birth. According to the latest research (Brown 1997), most babies who acquire a herpes infection from their mothers are born to women who first acquired genital herpes during the weeks immediately preceding labor and delivery. A woman infected at this point in gestation does not have time to develop a full immune response to HSV before delivery and thus is not able to transfer protective antibodies to her baby in the womb.

It should be noted that while women who become infected late in pregnancy may have obvious lesions, they may also shed virus asymptomatically. The risk to the baby is greatest when the recently infected mother is shedding virus asymptomatically at delivery. Without the warning sign of obvious genital lesions, the attending physician or midwife will have no reason to consider cesarean-section delivery.

Because genital herpes acquired in the third trimester poses the greatest risk to the baby, experts today recommend that women who are at risk for infection by either viral serotype — that is, women who are seronegative for HSV-1 and/or HSV-2— should either abstain from sexual intercourse or use condoms for intercourse in the final nine weeks of pregnancy. Such women should also be aware of the risk of acquiring an HSV-1 genital infection from cunnilingus from a partner with an oral HSV-1 infection.

Neonatal HSV infection is discussed in more detail in Section 2.9.

3.55 Pregnant, Diagnosed with Genital Herpes

Even a woman with long-standing genital herpes can transmit HSV infection to her baby. The risk is greatest if she has a symptomatic infection at the time of delivery. In such cases, cesarean section within four hours of the mother's water breaking is the recommended procedure.

If you are pregnant and have a history of frequent symptomatic recurrences, ask your doctor about the possibility of using suppressive antiviral therapy to reduce the risk of an outbreak. In such cases, suppressive therapy might be started only in the weeks leading up to and including delivery. Studies of suppressive antiviral therapy to reduce the need for cesarean delivery among women with genital herpes are now in progress.

The manufacturers of acyclovir have maintained a registry of babies born to women taking acyclovir, and to date, there have been no cases of fetal injury reported (Andrews 1992). (The registry does not represent a scientific study; participation is strictly voluntary on the part of the prescribing physician.) Acyclovir has not been linked with birth defects, but it's not as yet used routinely during pregnancy.

Neonatal HSV infection is discussed in more detail in Section 2.9.

3.6 The Drug Approval Process and Alternative Medicines

In some circles, an anti-scientific bias has taken root over the last 20 years with regard to health and medicine. One offshoot of this phenomenon has been the proliferation of natural, holistic, and alternative remedies for a broad assortment of diseases and chronic conditions. Herpes is no exception. You may encounter claims from those who market these products regarding their safety and effectiveness, but our advice is to be wary. These products are not regulated. You should be on guard against the herpes charlatans who claim to have a cure or a new treatment "never before available in this country." If you enroll in such a program, at best you are probably throwing away a considerable sum of money. At worst, you are risking serious injury from toxic side effects.

The only reliable way to determine whether a drug is safe and effective is to study it in **randomized, double-blind, placebo-controlled trials.** In such trials, patients are randomly assigned to receive either the active drug or a placebo (a visually identical but completely inactive substitute, a "sugar pill"). **Double-blind** means that neither the patients nor the doctors who monitor their well-being during the trial know who is taking the active drug and who is taking the placebo. This avoids bias in recording and interpreting the results. At the end of the study the outcomes for the two groups are compared. Presumably, any physiologic or medicinal effects seen among patients taking the drug that are not seen in the placebo group are due to the active ingredient in the drug. A placebo, by definition, produces no physiologic or medicinal effects whatsoever.

The problem with unregulated natural and holistic "medicines" is that they are almost never subjected to this kind of rigorous study. Maybe they work, maybe they don't. Maybe they're safe, maybe they're not. Without double-blind, randomized, placebo-controlled trials in a sufficient number of patients to establish the facts, there's simply no way to know if natural remedies have anything real to offer the herpes patient.

Many natural substances marketed as "alternative" medicines *are* in fact biologically active (a basic property of all medicines). They may even have medicinal qualities, but they may also produce side effects. Just because a substance occurs naturally doesn't mean it is automatically safe and devoid of side effects. Some of the most potent yet toxic drugs in our modern arsenal of anticancer agents are extracted from the periwinkle plant. Digitalis, an extract of the foxglove plant, is prescribed to millions of heart patients, but even a slight overdose can result in fatal disturbances in heart rhythm. And let's not forget that certain mushrooms are poisonous.

Because many so-called "natural" remedies are actually classified as herbs, spices, or nutritional supplements, they aren't subject to the same careful scrutiny the FDA applies to the drug industry. The safe dosing levels of these substances have never been determined through scientific study, so no one knows *how much* is *too much*. Almost any substance can be seriously toxic if consumed in sufficient quantities.

Every prescription drug sold in the United States goes through at least four levels of rigorous scientific study before it can be approved for general use:

- In the **preclinical phase,** the drug is given to laboratory animals to see if it has any tendency to cause birth defects or cancer and to determine the dose at which adverse effects begin to appear.
- In the second level of testing, which is actually designated **phase I,** the drug is usually given to fewer than 100 healthy human volunteers to study how it behaves in the body. *Is the drug safe? In which body tissues does it concentrate? Does it cross the blood-brain barrier? How long does it remain active in the body? How does the body eliminate it?*
- In **phase II,** the drug is given to 100–200 people who have the disease in question to determine the best dose and to confirm that the drug performs as expected.
- If the drug makes it out of phase II, in **phase III,** it is studied in hundreds to thousands of patients. Phase III studies are either placebo-controlled trials or double-blind randomized comparisons. Randomized comparisons are conducted to gauge how the drug performs at proposed recommended dose levels and to compare its performance with that of other drugs used to treat the same disease. Side effects are also examined more closely in phase III.

While a drug's average effectiveness and toxicity in the general population can be assessed by clinical studies, the results of those studies can only express statistical realities. For example: Drug A lowered the frequency of recurrent lesions in 95 percent of patients; Drug B caused headache in 12 percent of patients; etc. A clinical trial can tell us the odds that a drug will perform a certain way in any given patient, but whether or not the drug will work for you without producing unacceptable side effects can only be determined *empirically*— that is, by trial and error. The fact that a drug did or didn't work for someone else or caused a particular side effect in a friend, or a friend-of-a-friend, has nothing *whatsoever* to do with the performance of the drug in you. Beware of *anecdotal* evidence — stories. This applies to all manner of home remedies and alternative medicines, as well as to prescription and nonprescription drugs!

3.61 A Note on Lysine

A substantial number of people with herpes say they are able to reduce the frequency of recurrent episodes by augmenting their intake of **L-lysine** monohydrochloride, an amino acid that occurs naturally in a wide variety of foods. They propose a dietary approach to the management of herpes that emphasizes increased consumption of foods rich in lysine and decreased consumption of foods high in another amino acid, arginine. Proponents of this approach believe that lysine suppresses HSV while arginine promotes its expression. Interestingly, arginine is believed to enhance the body's immune function, which raises the question of whether its reduction in the diet may increase one's susceptibility to nonherpetic infection.

According to the American Social Health Association, a few small studies have shown a clinical benefit associated with high doses of lysine taken orally as a supplement to the lysine consumed in the normal diet. However, other studies, including a 1984 trial by the National Institutes of Health, failed to detect any therapeutic benefit.

No safe dose range for lysine has ever been established by conventional clinical methodology. Because of this, and because the most thorough study to date found no therapeutic value in lysine, the author and editors of this book urge any person with herpes who wants to have the maximum impact on HSV to consider proven antiviral medications before dietary supplements. Based on available data, the use of lysine to control recurrent episodes of genital herpes cannot be recommended. In addition, lysine has not been proven effective against asymptomatic viral shedding—a serious issue.

3.7 Genital Herpes in the New Millennium

What is being done to end the epidemic of genital herpes? HSV research is by no means at a standstill. Recent years have seen the introduction of a new generation of effective antiviral drugs, including valacyclovir and famciclovir. But many are still wondering: Where is the drug that will suppress latent virus completely and prevent recurrences and asymptomatic shedding once and for all? Where is the vaccine that will keep future generations from contracting genital herpes? And where is the cure, which will rid the body of the virus?

The easiest of those questions to address is the last one. Most experts agree, barring a totally unexpected breakthrough, any cure for herpes is many years away. Pessimism in this area is mainly due to the nature of HSV latency. HSV acquired through genital infection establishes latency in the **sacral ganglia,** bundles of nerve cells at the base of the spine. The task is to find a way to kill virus without killing nerve cells. Currently available antivirals, which are very effective against replicating HSV in skin cells at genital sites, have generally been considered useless against latent (or dormant) virus in the sacral ganglia. In essence, these drugs depend on chemical signals from actively replicating virus to tell them which skin cells to attack. Research is still ongoing into the potential effect of antivirals on latent HSV. In one experimental animal model, latency was prevented by treating laboratory mice with famciclovir within 22 hours of infection. It's unclear whether or how this finding applies to humans.

Dormant virus in the sacral ganglia does not replicate; it exists in a much reduced metabolic state. And although we have identified one or two of the genes that remain "switched on" in dormant HSV, we have not been able to identify the constituent proteins of those genes. Until we identify those proteins, we can't even develop an assay to *look for* a drug that will get into the neuron and block them.

Historically, from a public health perspective, the most successful disease prevention efforts have used vaccines. Although herpes is not high on the National Institute of Medicine's list of diseases for which vaccines are needed, a reasonable scientific effort is being made to find one. The effort is modest, however, given the magnitude of the epidemic. At the time of this writing, at least seven experimental vaccines were in various stages of clinical development. An eighth, Chiron Corporation's recombinant protein vaccine, had just been abandoned because, in the final phase of clinical testing (phase III), it proved ineffective.

One of the problems in creating an effective vaccine for genital herpes is that the two most tried and true methods of development have significant problems. One of the traditional ways to make a vaccine is to chemically deactivate a virus and administer this deactivated version to boost immunity. The current flu or Salk polio vaccines take this approach. For HSV, however, researchers have been extremely cautious with this approach because it leaves large amounts of HSV DNA in the preparation, and some HSV genes can cause human cells to undergo uncontrolled growth. In short, the fear has been that inoculating people with large amounts of HSV DNA may cause cancer. As research has proceeded over the years, the carcinogenic potential of HSV DNA has become less of a concern, but unfortunately the vaccines developed from deactivated virus have not been very successful in laboratory animals.

Another approach has involved the use of live virus weakened by the removal of certain genes we think are important in transmission. This weakened or "attenuated" form of HSV is presumably less likely to cause symptomatic infection. The problem here is that we would be introducing into the human body a live virus that replicates and colonizes the nervous system. Will it remain forever attenuated or will it mutate and become as virulent as normal HSV? If a person becomes immunosuppressed later in life, will the attenuated virus cause problems? One attenuated HSV vaccine did enter clinical trials, but it caused too many side effects, and its development was put on hold until a safer agent emerges. (*An interesting side note:* Attenuated HSV is being investigated as a vehicle to deliver anticancer drugs to brain tumors, precisely because of its ability to invade the nervous system.)

Thus, scientists are using genetic engineering to develop new approaches. Some are using pieces of HSV DNA (DNA vaccines); others are purifying various proteins of the virus and using these proteins (subunits) as vaccine candidates. Several of these are under investigation now. In addition, a better understanding of the immune response to herpes is likely to boost vaccine research efforts.

At present, vaccine development and the search for more effective antivirals (drugs that can boost the immune response and keep the virus "quiet" in the nervous system) are the major avenues of HSV research.

part

FOUR

CYNTHIA'S STORY
Epilogue

～

Dr. Foster didn't see Cynthia again until the following May, when she came in for her annual Pap smear. She had cut her hair and appeared to be very happy. He assumed the apparent good mood and cheerful affect were related to her upcoming wedding, so he asked whether their plans were still moving forward.

"I was going to tell you later," she said, laughing. "Brian and I broke up in January. I left him."

Dr. Foster was clearly surprised at this news and eager to hear the details. "What happened, if you don't mind my asking?"

"Well," Cynthia began, "just after New Year's, Brian and I decided to go to Montreal for a short vacation. There's a beautiful rolling wooded area outside town where we went cross-country skiing the year we met. Brian thought it would be nice to go back before the wedding.

"Anyway. We were skiing for a couple of days, and then we spent a couple of days in Montreal, shopping and just hanging out. It's one of my favorite places in the world.

"Our second day in town, Brian had something he wanted to do. I don't remember what it was, but I didn't feel like going. I had a terrible sinus headache, and all I wanted to do was take a nap. So he went out, wherever, I don't remember. I stayed in the room. I hadn't brought any kind of aspirin or antihistamines or anything with me, so I looked in Brian's shaving kit. I found a brown plastic pill bottle with no label and opened it, hoping to find aspirin or ibuprofen or something, but instead, guess what?"

Dr. Foster shook his head and shrugged his shoulders.

"I'll give you a hint," Cynthia said. "Pale blue capsules, with a little black unicorn on them."

"Acyclovir?"

"Exactamundo," Cynthia laughed, making an "okay" sign with her thumb and index finger.

"A genuine mystery. Please continue."

Cynthia clearly enjoyed telling the story. "I thought it was pretty weird. Then I thought, *'Well, maybe he's keeping some on hand in case he catches it from me,'* you know? But it's a prescription drug. How would he get a prescription for it? Yadda yadda yadda . . .

"Anyway, I put the capsules back. Then I did something really sneaky. Later that afternoon when he got back to the room, I told him I thought I felt another infection coming on, but I didn't have my medicine with me, and I was really scared. I laid it on thick, too — sniffling and pretending to be on the verge of tears — but he volunteered nothing, not a word.

"He actually suggested that I call *you,* to see if you could phone in my prescription to a pharmacy in Montreal. He even asked me if I wanted to go home early."

"This is incredible," Dr. Foster sighed.

"There's more," Cynthia said. "I waited a minute, then I excused myself. I said I needed to blow my nose, and I went to the bathroom. When I came back out, I tossed the brown pill bottle on the bed and said, very calmly, 'I guess these would do, but what's the expiration date?'"

Dr. Foster laughed.

"At first he was angry," Cynthia continued, "I allowed him about a millisecond's outrage over my 'snooping' in his shaving kit — can you believe that, 'snooping'? Then I cut him off cold and demanded an explanation. He broke down totally. *And this you will not believe.* It turns out he's had herpes for at least ten years."

"No!"

"Oh yeah," Cynthia said, nodding emphatically. "He knew he had it all along. He said he didn't tell me when we first met, and I quote, because he *'wasn't sure this was going anywhere'*. But, he says, he really did fall in love with me, and he was afraid that if I found out he had herpes, I'd leave him. He was too afraid to tell me. He said he tried to be careful so I wouldn't get it. He had a very mild case, only one or two outbreaks each year. They only lasted a few days, and he was always able to avoid actual intercourse with me until they cleared up. Seems someone told him, years ago, that you're not contagious if you don't have lesions."

"Well, that explains a lot, doesn't it?" Dr. Foster said, looking down at his feet and shaking his head slowly. "So all this was just too much for you?"

"Well, believe it or not, no. At least, not at first. I really felt sorry for him at first. I mean he was crying like a baby by the end of it, and begging me to forgive him. We were out of town, after all. What are you going to do?

"But when we got back, the more I thought about it, the more furious I got. I mean, for how long was he 'not sure this was going anywhere,' anyway? That's not the way I remember it. That's not the sort of thing he was saying to me when we first started dating. And then the lie — the not telling me — and then what I went through with that first episode. To tell you the truth, I'm not sure what I would have done if he'd told me when we first met. I want to believe I would have risen above my fear —I was so smitten back then. Maybe I would have gotten herpes anyway, maybe not, but the more I thought about it the madder I became, and after three weeks of simmering rage, I just snapped. I left him, and moved in with a girl from work who needed a roommate. I've been looking around for a place of my own. But we get along. I'm not in any big hurry."

Dr. Foster just smiled and shook his head in disbelief.

"There's more," Cynthia said, excitedly. "I've met someone else."

"So soon? That's great."

"Yeah," Cynthia said, dreamily, "I wasn't even looking. I was like,

'Men! Who needs 'em?' And out of the blue there's this guy at work. When he heard Brian and I had split up, he started asking me out, and he simply would not take no for an answer." Cynthia actually giggled at this point, "He's five years younger than me and incredibly sweet."

~

Cynthia had asked Dr. Foster earlier if she could have a moment in private after the examination to discuss something, and when she finished getting dressed, she was escorted to his office by the nurse who had assisted with the examination. A few minutes later, Dr. Foster came in and closed the door. "I have to ask," he said, as he took his seat behind the desk, "but you don't have to answer. Have you told your new guy about your herpes?"

"I told Paul the second or third time we went out — I don't remember — but it was weeks before we ever slept together. He asked me about my break-up with Brian, so I told him the whole story. He's okay with it. He is concerned about getting herpes — who wouldn't be, especially after I told him about my initial experience? — but he says I'm worth it."

"I'm honestly not all that surprised," Dr. Foster said. "Some guys can handle it, some can't. What sort of precautions are you taking?"

"Condoms, but we'd be doing that anyway, at least until we've both been tested for HIV. He wants to be tested for herpes also, and that's what I wanted to ask you about. I told him about type-specific blood tests and how so many people are infected without ever knowing they have herpes. He figures if we're going to be together, we should at least find out if he has HSV-2 antibodies. If he does, that's one less thing to worry about."

Dr. Foster jotted down a name and a telephone number on a slip of paper and handed it to Cynthia. "Here's a thought," he said. "We've closed enrollment here at the Clinic, but one of my colleagues across town is starting to accept couples for that vaccine study we discussed back in the fall. If Paul tests negative for HSV-2, you might think about participating. If you decide to pursue it, call this guy. Tell him you're a patient of mine and that I referred you. Otherwise, if Paul needs more information or some help lining up a blood test, tell him to call me. I already like him. He sounds like a keeper."

"I think so," Cynthia said, rising to leave. She shook hands with Dr. Foster.

"I still can't get over your story," he said, "but I'm glad things worked out as well as they did. You've been through some changes."

"In a lot of ways, yes." Cynthia mused, pausing in the doorway. "You know? I wouldn't wish the experience on anyone, but it's not the end of the world either. In a lot of ways, I'm happier than I've ever been. And when I think about Brian and last September . . . it all seems like another world."

~

That same evening, around 7 p.m., at a trendy uptown watering hole, a handsome attorney named Brian approaches the bar. He takes a seat next to an attractive young woman in a stylish blue suit, orders a dry martini, and in a credible Scottish brogue adds, "Shaken, not stirred."

His drink arrives. He takes a sip, then turns to the young woman in blue and says, "I can tell right away we have a lot in common."

Twenty minutes later he's buying the drinks, and quoting dialogue from *The Godfather.*

Turns out they both like a lot of the same movies.

And he loves Thai food as much as she does — *what are the odds?*

"Say, listen, have you had dinner?" he asks, enthusiastically, and starts telling her about a hot new restaurant in the Village that he's been dying to try.

"No kidding!" She's seen an article about it in *New York* magazine, even knows the name.

"The owner is a client of mine," he says, casually. "I've been meaning to check it out, whaddya say, my treat?"

It's a first date right out of Hollywood. A hot new restaurant in the Village. The wine and the laughter. The intense conversation and the cab ride home. But in time, just one more tearful patient asking her doctor, "How? Why?"

chapter four

GENITAL HERPES:
QUESTIONS AND ANSWERS

~

The information presented thus far covers in a systematic way most of the topics that concern those with genital herpes. Sometimes, however, the systematic approach leaves unanswered the subtleties of a particular question. This section is intended to answer directly some of the most frequently asked questions about genital herpes — and in doing so to review some of the material in earlier chapters.

⬦ *I think I might have genital herpes. How can I be sure? What are the symptoms?*

If you think you have genital herpes and want to confirm it, the best thing you can do is see a doctor or a health care provider experienced in sexually transmitted diseases. The diagnosis is not always straightforward and can baffle even a trained physician. Recurrent episodes, which are generally milder than first episodes, can be especially hard to recognize, but first episodes often go unrecognized as well. Symptoms may be subtle or may resemble those of other diseases and conditions. Genital herpes can mimic many other sexually transmitted diseases in appearance. Mild lesions may also be mistaken for eczema, psoriasis, pimples, jock itch, an allergic rash, or an ingrown hair. Laboratory tests (viral culture; type-specific serology) to confirm a diagnosis of genital herpes are highly recommended, and you should see a practitioner who has access to such tests.

Diagnosis is easiest during a symptomatic initial episode of infection. Local symptoms are likely to include a rash-like eruption in the genital area. This typically progresses to the formation of clear fluid-filled bumps on an area of reddened skin (the classic description is "dew drops on a rose petal"). The vesicles tend to become larger and more blister-like, eventually rupturing and then scabbing or crusting over. On mucosal surfaces, such as the inner surface of the vagina, lesions are more likely to appear as ulcers. The lesions of first-episode genital herpes are usually quite painful. Women may have a profuse, watery vaginal discharge; men may have a clear discharge from the urethra. Associated local symptoms may include painful urination and painful defecation due to lesions in the urethra and rectal areas. The possible constitutional symptoms of first-episode genital herpes include fever, headache, malaise (a vague feeling of bodily discomfort), muscle aches, anorexia (loss of appetite), and painful swollen lymph nodes in the groin and pelvic areas. Recurrent episodes tend to be milder than the initial episode.

See the following section(s) for additional information: 2.5 Symptoms.

◇ *Why do so few people with genital herpes have symptoms?*

It appears to be largely a question of immunity. Some people have better natural and/or acquired defenses against HSV infection. However, what may be a more accurate way of framing the issue is to say that most people with genital herpes don't have *recognizable* symptoms. The public has been told for many years that genital herpes always produces severe symptoms. As a result, people with subtle signs and symptoms don't think to ask themselves, "Could this be herpes?" It has been shown that when people with supposedly asymptomatic herpes are trained to recognize the subtler signs and symptoms of disease, many are able to identify when they are having an outbreak.

◈ *How could I have genital herpes? I've been in an exclusive relationship for years. I trust my partner. I haven't been fooling around. And neither of us had herpes when we met.*

The sudden appearance of genital herpes in a presumably monogamous relationship does not necessarily mean one partner has been unfaithful.

How you got genital herpes is a pretty easy question to answer. Genital herpes is transmitted during sexual intercourse (vaginal or anal) and during oral sex. Admittedly, there are other possibilities. **Autoinoculation** is the transmission of HSV infection from one part of the body to another and can occur during a symptomatic primary infection, when large amounts of virus are present and the body has not had adequate time to develop a full immune response. Autoinoculation could involve transmission of HSV-1 from the mouth to a finger. It could involve transmission of HSV-1, by hand, from the mouth to the genitals. While we know that autoinoculation *can* occur, it is very seldom (if ever) the cause of genital herpes, most cases of which are due to HSV-2.

When you got genital herpes is another question altogether. Either you or your partner could have had it for years without knowing. The vast majority of genital HSV infections produce no recognized symptoms, yet these silently recurring infections are fully capable of delivering infectious virus to genital surfaces even though no rash or other lesions are visible. It is possible that you acquired your current infection recently when your partner was shedding virus asymptomatically. Another possibility is that you are experiencing the first symptomatic recurrence of an infection you actually acquired some time ago. Remember: Herpes simplex virus can lie low, undetected for years; then, for reasons we don't understand, it can begin producing recurrent symptomatic infections. However, if your symptoms are quite severe, there is a good chance you are experiencing a primary (first) infection. Timely blood testing can confirm this, as your HSV serostatus shifts from negative to positive.

See the following section(s) for additional information: 1.52 HSV-2 Transmission; 1.6 How HSV Infection Is Established.

⟨?⟩ *How often will my infection recur and cause symptoms?*

It's not possible to predict what any one person's experience will be. Statistically speaking, about 90 percent of people with a symptomatic first episode of genital herpes will have at least one recurrence in the following year. On average, genital herpes caused by HSV-1 recurs about once a year, and genital herpes caused by HSV-2 recurs about four times a year. However, some patients may have 12 or more recurrences a year while others have none. Each person's experience of genital herpes is unique. Consider keeping a diary to record prodromal symptoms and recurrences. Learning your prodromal symptoms can help you recognize outbreaks before they occur. The diary is also a convenient place to write down questions you want to ask your doctor at subsequent visits.

See the following section(s) for more information: 2.54 Prodromal Symptoms; 2.6 Patterns of Recurrence.

⟨?⟩ *Will it ever go away?*

If you mean, "will the virus ever leave your body?" the answer is no. Medical science has yet to find a way to rid the body of latent HSV-1 or HSV-2. But if you mean, "will the infection stop recurring?" the answer is a cautiously qualified maybe. In many people, the frequency of recurrences declines over the years. In some, recurrent outbreaks disappear completely for long periods of time, although spontaneous reactivation is always a possibility. Asymptomatic viral shedding probably continues, even after symptomatic recurrences have stopped, which means the risk of transmission persists even in the absence of rash and lesions. Antiviral therapy can dramatically reduce the frequency of asymptomatic shedding.

See the following section(s) for more information: 1.62 Latency, Reactivation, and Recurrence; 2.6 Patterns of Recurrence.

⟨?⟩ *What triggers recurrences?*

This is one of the more poorly understood aspects of HSV infection. In their efforts to devise vaccines and new treatments for herpes, scientists are trying to find the answer at a microbiologic level.

A number of physical stimuli are reported to trigger recurrent episodes of infection, including sunburn, surgery causing trauma to the area surrounding the infected nerve roots (ganglia), and irritation to the genital area (even the friction of rigorous intercourse). Many people with herpes report that recurrences are triggered by increased stress in their lives, but this effect has not been confirmed scientifically.

With time, most people learn to recognize their own pattern of recurrence, but don't assume you'll be able to predict every outbreak.

◈ How long do the symptoms of recurrent infection last?

Recurrent infections tend to be of shorter duration than primary or nonprimary first episodes. It varies from person to person, and episode to episode. On average, complete healing of lesions has been reported in seven to ten days in the published research, although many outbreaks will heal in less than a week. Recurrent infections also tend to be less severe than initial episodes. Constitutional symptoms (e.g., fever, headache, stiff neck, swollen lymph nodes) are uncommon during recurrent episodes, and lesions (rash, sores, etc.) tend to concentrate on one side of the genitals. Ulcers on mucocutaneous surfaces rarely occur.

See the following section(s) for more information: 2.5 Symptoms; 2.53 Symptomatic Recurrent Genital Herpes.

◈ How often does a person with genital herpes shed virus asymptomatically?

Asymptomatic viral shedding is an important concern. The presence of infectious virus on genital surfaces in the absence of symptoms is far more common than we once thought. As recently as five years ago, we would have said asymptomatic shedding occurs only one day in every hundred; however, recent research using a supersensitive diagnostic technique called polymerase chain reaction suggests the true frequency of asymptomatic viral shedding may be closer to one day in every five. This finding has important implications for the prevention of transmission and helps explain the fact that up to 70 percent of new cases of genital herpes are acquired from a partner with no signs or symptoms of infection at the time.

The frequency of asymptomatic shedding is related to the frequency of symptomatic recurrence: people with low rates of symptomatic recurrences have far fewer episodes of asymptomatic shedding than people with frequent symptomatic outbreaks. People with genital herpes caused by HSV-1 shed virus less frequently than those with an infection caused by HSV-2.

See the following section(s) for more information: 3.42 Suppressive Antiviral Therapy for Recurrent Genital Herpes.

◇ *Are there drugs available to get rid of herpes?*

No — nor are there any natural, holistic, or other alternative remedies that can get rid of herpes. Despite what you may hear or read to the contrary, there is no known cure for genital herpes. No one knows how to eliminate or permanently deactivate latent HSV-1 or HSV-2.

There are three highly effective antiviral drugs available to help control genital herpes: acyclovir, famciclovir, and valacyclovir. The latter two, which were developed more recently, offer therapeutic advantages over acyclovir. Acyclovir, on the other hand is available in generic form and may be significantly less expensive than the newer drugs. Your doctor will prescribe the one he or she thinks is right for you.

The inability of the three currently available antiviral drugs to eliminate latent virus is due to their mechanism of action. All three drugs are selectively taken up by and activated in cells that contain replicating virus. Once HSV has established latency in the cells of the nerve root (ganglia), it stops replicating — becomes silent, so to speak — and the antiviral drugs don't know it's there.

See the following section(s): 3.2 Antiviral Therapy: What It Can and Can't Do; 3.6 The Drug Approval Process and Alternative Medicines.

◇ *What is episodic therapy?*

Episodic therapy relies on your ability to recognize the early warning symptoms of genital herpes, the prodromal symptoms. At the first appearance of prodromal symptoms, you initiate antiviral therapy. This early intervention can reduce the severity of a recurrent episode or, in some cases, prevent it from progressing to a fully symptomatic state.

Obviously, episodic therapy requires that you have a supply of antiviral drug on hand at all times. Episodic therapy has no effect on the frequency of recurrences.

Episodic therapy with valacyclovir appears to be superior to that with acyclovir in aborting recurrent outbreaks.

See the following section(s) for more information: 3.41 Episodic Antiviral Therapy for Recurrent Genital Herpes.

◇ *What are the uses of suppressive antiviral therapy?*

Suppressive therapy means you take an antiviral drug every day; suppressive therapy with acyclovir can dramatically reduce the frequency of recurrent episodes for most patients and eliminate outbreaks completely for others. Suppressive therapy with acyclovir has also been shown to reduce the frequency of asymptomatic viral shedding by up to 94 percent. It's logical to assume that such a substantial reduction in the number of days of viral shedding would also reduce the risk of transmission. Studies to test this hypothesis in discordant couples (couples in which only one member is infected) are now underway. Transmission is a key issue for many couples. It is especially important for couples in which only the husband is infected and the wife is pregnant or intends to become pregnant. We are increasingly looking to suppressive antiviral therapy as a way to reduce the risk, regardless of the frequency or severity of the infected partner's recurrences.

The initial studies on reducing asymptomatic viral shedding with suppressive therapy used acyclovir. A more recent study using valacyclovir found equivalent results (Wald 1998), and valacyclovir is the drug being used in the transmission studies mentioned above.

See the following section(s) for more information: 3.42 Suppressive Antiviral Therapy for Recurrent Genital Herpes; 3.5 Prevention.

◇ *Are antiviral drugs safe, and do they have unpleasant short- or long-term side effects?*

The real safety profile of a drug can only be determined over time. The more people who take the drug without experiencing dangerous side effects, the safer the drug is presumed to be.

All three of the currently approved antivirals can be regarded as safe for their approved uses because they have completed the FDA-required testing for those uses. However, neither famciclovir nor valacyclovir has been in use long enough to make the same long-term safety claims as acyclovir. Acyclovir has been used in more than 30 million people since 1978 with no serious side effects reported. No serious safety problems have been reported with famciclovir or valacyclovir either, but the collected experience with both is comparatively limited. In the body, valacyclovir is converted into acyclovir and other metabolites, and the long-term safety record of valacyclovir is expected to be as good as that of acyclovir. Over time, famciclovir may prove equally safe. The adverse events reported with all three drugs are relatively infrequent and generally mild. You're unlikely to have a problem tolerating any of the three.

See the following section(s) for more information: 3.3 Treating the First Symptomatic Episode; 3.41 Episodic Antiviral Therapy for Recurrent Genital Herpes (Table 3.41).

◇ *How expensive are antiviral drugs?*

In preparing this book, we conducted a telephone survey of five major pharmacies in Durham, NC, asking the cost of 30 acyclovir (Zovirax®) capsules, 30 famciclovir (Famvir®) tablets, and 30 valacyclovir (Valtrex®) caplets. Prices varied considerably, and no one outlet had the lowest price for all three drugs. Using the U.S. Centers for Disease Control's dosing guidelines and based on our survey, the average cost for one year of suppressive therapy ranged from just under $1,000 per year to more than $2,000 per year. However, the antiviral market is changing.

In the months since our initial survey, patent protection on acyclovir has lapsed, and a number of generic manufacturers have entered the market. Generic drugs are almost always less expensive than the branded versions. Also, at press time for this book, the prices of valacyclovir and famciclovir were fluctuating. The best advice we can give you is to shop around, and be sure to find out what your Managed Care Organization, HMO, or insurer is willing to reimburse.

When selecting antiviral therapy, consider not just the price of the drug, but also its *value*. While valacyclovir and famciclovir may be more expensive than generic acyclovir, they also offer therapeutic advantages such as less frequent dosing.

◇ *Can condoms prevent transmission?*

Condoms may reduce the risk of transmission between symptomatic outbreaks, but they cannot eliminate the risk completely, any more than they can prevent pregnancy 100 percent of the time. Condoms can break or slip off during intercourse. More of an issue, however, is that while condoms cover most of the penis, they do not cover other areas from which virus could be shed if lesions were present. It is also conceivable that uncovered skin in the male genital area could be vulnerable to infection from virus in vaginal secretions.

See the following section(s) for more information: 3.5 Prevention.

◇ *Can suppressive therapy prevent transmission?*

Whether suppressive therapy can prevent transmission is not known for certain. We presume it can. We know suppressive therapy can reduce asymptomatic viral shedding, which is responsible for up to 70 percent of new cases of genital herpes. In one study, suppressive therapy reduced the number of days of asymptomatic shedding by 94 percent, and most experts agree that such a dramatic reduction in viral shedding should correlate with a reduced risk of transmission. Ongoing studies will put this hypothesis to the test.

See the following section(s) for more information: 3.42 Suppressive Antiviral Therapy for Recurrent Genital Herpes; 3.5 Prevention.

◇ *Does oral sex pose less risk of transmission than regular intercourse?*

The risk of HSV transmission during oral sex is substantial. It is the major way in which genital HSV-1 infection is acquired, and HSV-1 accounts for a growing percentage of genital herpes. Oral HSV-2 infection can be acquired through oral sex with a partner who has genital herpes. Genital HSV-2 infection, on the other hand, is rarely acquired through oral sex, chiefly because oral HSV-2 infections recur so infrequently.

Remember that HSV infection occurs most easily when virus comes in direct contact with a mucosal surface, like the lining of the mouth or vagina. A woman with genital herpes who wants to avoid transmitting the virus to her partner during oral sex can use barrier protection — a latex dental dam, a cut condom, or kitchen plastic wrap — to physically isolate her genitals from her partner's mouth. A man with genital herpes who wants to avoid transmitting the virus to his partner during oral sex can wear a condom. The same precautions can be taken to reduce the risk of transmission of HSV-1 or HSV-2 from mouth to genitals.

We know that after the initial episode, oral HSV-2 infections recur less frequently than oral HSV-1 infections, and genital HSV-1 infections recur less frequently than genital HSV-2 infections. Fewer recurrences mean fewer opportunities for transmission, but the risk is still real.

See the following section(s) for more information: 3.5 Prevention; 1.5 How HSV Infection Is Transmitted; 2.21 HSV-1 or HSV-2?

◈ *How can I tell if my prospective sexual partner has herpes?*

You can't always tell, but don't overlook the obvious. Given that an oral HSV infection in your partner can become a genital infection in you through oral sex, you should avoid receiving oral sex from someone who has a cold sore or fever blister on or around his or her lips. If you are able to inspect the genital area of a prospective partner, any type of rash, sore, or ulceration should, at the very least, give you pause. Even if it isn't genital herpes, it could be another sexually transmitted disease.

You can always ask. We live in an age when sexually transmitted disease is a matter of life and death. If you're contemplating a sexual relationship with a new partner, you most certainly should discuss past sexual experiences and sexually transmitted diseases — *first*. As long as you're talking about AIDS, you might as well talk about herpes. But remember, most people who have genital herpes never experience obvious symptoms. The best way to know for sure, therefore, is for you and your partner to get one of the new type-specific blood tests. (See Appendix B.)

If you are frequently having sex with people you don't really know and with whom you have not had an in-depth "safer sex" discussion, the proper use of condoms, plastic wrap, and dental dams will offer you some protection from herpes.

If you are having *unprotected sex* with people you don't really know, you are literally gambling with your life, and herpes could be the least of your worries.

See the following section(s) for more information: 3.5 Prevention; 2.73 Testing for HSV.

◈ *If a person already has genital herpes, can he or she become reinfected?*

This phenomenon, reinfection with a different strain of the same HSV serotype, is called *exogenous reinfection.* It has been seen in people whose immune response is compromised or suppressed (AIDS patients, burn victims, organ transplant recipients). But in people with normal immune systems, exogenous reinfection is extremely unlikely. It is also unlikely that a person with genital herpes due to HSV-2 could develop a second infection due to HSV-1, because HSV-2 confers a great deal of immunity against HSV-1. The reverse is less true, though HSV-1, as we have discussed, does confer partial immunity to HSV-2.

See the following section(s) for more information: 1.7 The Antigenic Connection Between HSV-1 and HSV-2.

◈ *I'm subject to frequently recurring cold sores; do cold sores give you immunity to genital herpes?*

Remember that there are two types of herpes simplex virus — HSV-1 and HSV-2 — and that both viruses can cause infection at oral and genital sites. The degree of immunity you have to infection with either herpesvirus depends on your previous exposure. If your cold sores are due to HSV-1, it is highly unlikely that you could be reinfected with HSV-1 at another anatomical site. Previous infection with HSV-1 may reduce the risk of acquiring HSV-2, although it cannot prevent it. Previous infection with HSV-1 also tends to moderate the severity of subsequent HSV-2 infection. Conversely, previous infection with HSV-2 tends to moderate the severity of subsequent infection with HSV-1. If your cold sores are due to HSV-2, it is highly unlikely that you could ever be reinfected with HSV-2 at another site, including the genitals, but you would still face a small chance of infection with HSV-1.

HSV-1 "prefers" oral sites; HSV-2 "prefers" genital sites. Recurrence rates for both viruses are higher at the preferred sites. The fact that you describe your cold sores as "frequently recurring" suggests your oral infection is due to HSV-1. That being the case, you are highly unlikely to acquire a genital infection due to HSV-1, but are still vulnerable to genital infection with HSV-2.

◇ *I'm a gay woman who has been in a stable relationship for over a year. I've heard STDs are not much of a problem among lesbians. I don't worry much about HIV, but I do get occasional cold sores. I worry I might give my partner herpes, even though I only have outbreaks about twice a year. Is there anything we can do to prevent this from happening?*

The most realistic precaution you can take is avoid mouth kissing, oral-genital, or oral-anal contact during an outbreak of cold sores, including the prodromal period of numbness or tingling you may experience immediately prior to an outbreak. Asymptomatic shedding of HSV between symptomatic outbreaks occurs at oral sites, just as it does at genital sites, and its frequency is related to the frequency of symptomatic outbreaks. However, it isn't really possible to estimate the risk to your partner.

There are precautions you can take to minimize the risk of oral-to-genital transmission (a latex dental dam, kitchen plastic wrap, or a cut condom placed between your mouth and your partner's genitals). However, let's try to put this issue in perspective. No one is going to suggest that every time you kiss your partner's mouth, you first slap a piece of plastic wrap over your own mouth. Extrapolating that same level of precaution to your oral-genital love-making may seem just as overcautious, especially in a long-term relationship. Your partner should at least be made aware that oral HSV infection can be transmitted to the genitals and perianal areas by oral sex. Whether you want to sacrifice a high degree of intimacy to further reduce what may already be a minimal risk of transmission is something for the two of you to decide, as a couple.

You could perhaps buy yourselves some peace of mind if you both have a Western blot serologic test performed to determine your antibody status (Cost: approx. $100). Assuming that your cold sores are caused by HSV-1, if your partner already has antibodies to HSV-1, you could stop worrying about infecting her. If your cold sores are due to HSV-2 (which is highly unlikely) and your partner has no antibodies to HSV-2, the risk of transmission is there.

It's worth noting that the majority of women who have sex with women also have a history of sex with men, and genital herpes can be transmitted between women through any sexual activity that brings the genital tissues and secretions of one partner in direct contact with the genitals of another, including the use of sexual devices. To prevent infections such as HSV and even hepatitis B, sex toys should be washed with alcohol or soap and water and thoroughly dried with a clean towel.

◈ *How do I tell my partner I have genital herpes, and what should I say?*

Telling a prospective partner you have herpes is probably easiest in the context of a more inclusive safer-sex conversation. Before you become involved with anyone sexually, you deserve to know something of his or her sexual history. *You* have information to share; perhaps he or she does, too.

Choose a quiet, private place with a relaxed atmosphere and try to ensure that you have ample time for discussion. It's normal to feel apprehensive about telling, and it will be normal for your partner to feel apprehensive about the possibility of contracting genital herpes. Remember that most people have a poor understanding of what genital herpes is, how common it is, how it is transmitted, and how it is treated.

Be prepared to answer questions, and don't expect your partner to come to terms with the issue on the spot. Give him or her time to take it all in. The following checklist offers some key points for discussion:

1. Genital herpes is a sexually transmitted disease caused by either HSV-1 or HSV-2. Most genital herpes is HSV-2; most oral herpes (cold sores, fever blisters) is HSV-1; but either virus can cause infection at either site.

2. Both herpes simplex viruses establish permanent latent infections which may recur periodically.

3. Genital herpes is a very common disease. Some 45,000,000 people in this country — roughly one in four over the age of 12 years — are infected with HSV-2, and roughly one million people become newly infected each year.

4. The main reason genital herpes is so widespread is that most of the people who are infected have subtle symptoms or no symptoms at all. They simply don't know they have the disease. In the most recent report of the National Health and Nutrition Examination Survey (1988–1994), less than 10 percent of those participants who tested positive for HSV-2 knew they had genital herpes. However, properly instructed, 50 percent or more of people with HSV infection previously deemed asymptomatic can learn to identify their symptoms.

5. Genital herpes cannot be cured. The virus cannot be eliminated from the body. (For perspective, you might mention that chickenpox and mononucleosis are also caused by human herpesviruses, and they also establish permanent latent infections. They're just a great deal less likely to recur.)

6. Genital herpes is highly treatable with antiviral therapy.

7. Suppressive antiviral therapy can dramatically reduce the frequency of recurrent infections — both symptomatic and asymptomatic.

8. Recurrent infections tend to be considerably milder than the initial episode of infection, and the frequency and severity of recurrences tends to lessen over time.

9. Without the consistent use of condoms, the average risk of transmission for couples in which only one partner has genital herpes is 10 percent per year. The risk for women in such couples may be as high as 15 percent; the risk for men, as low as 4 percent.

10. To minimize the risk of transmission, couples should refrain from sexual intercourse and oral sex during symptomatic recurrences and consider the use of condoms and other forms of barrier protection between symptomatic outbreaks. However, condoms do not offer complete protection. Antiviral therapy may also reduce the risk of transmission.

11. The most serious complication of genital herpes is infection of the newborn (neonatal HSV infection). If symptoms are present at the time of delivery, cesarean section is recommended; otherwise, a normal vaginal delivery is standard procedure. The greatest risk is when the mother contracts genital herpes in the third trimester and is shedding virus asymptomatically at the time of delivery.

chapter five

ADDITIONAL RESOURCES

~

5.1 HOTLINES

Sexual Health Communications Hotline   (888) 238-4238

Information specialists can refer you to a clinic in your area that specializes in the treatment of genital herpes or to clinics recruiting patients for clinical trials on a variety of sexual health concerns. Free videos and other educational materials are also available.

National Herpes Hotline   (919) 361-8488 (not toll-free)
(Mon–Fri, 9 a.m.–7 p.m., EST)

A service of the American Social Health Association (ASHA), this confidential hotline is staffed by trained counselors who will answer your questions about genital herpes or refer you to appropriate alternative sources. The service is touch-tone activated. Free publications are available, which will be mailed to you in a confidential envelope.

ASHA Resource Center   (800) 230-6039

A toll-free, touch-tone–activated service of the ASHA's Herpes Resource Center that allows you to leave your name and address to receive an information packet on genital herpes and other STDs, mailed to you at no charge in a confidential envelope.

National STD Hotline (800) 227-8922

This information hotline is operated by the U.S. Centers for Disease Control. Services include free printed information on genital herpes and other STDs and referral to a local public clinic for examination and treatment.

Sexually Transmitted Disease Information and Referral Center Hotline (800) 653-4325

A toll-free, touch-tone–activated service of the ASHA's Herpes Resource Center providing recorded information on genital herpes and other STDs. You can choose to speak with a counselor at any time during the recorded presentations. The system also allows you to enter your fax number for direct receipt of printed information on genital herpes and other STDs.

5.2 PUBLICATIONS/VIDEOS

Managing Herpes: How to Live and Love with a Chronic STD
Charles Ebel
$19.95

This illustrated 235-page paperback book addresses all aspects of genital herpes that are of importance to patients and their partners: from diagnosis and treatment of the initial episodes, to the management of recurrent infection, to the emotional and psychological dimensions of life with genital herpes. It includes useful information on legal issues and insurance questions. The author is a former director of the American Social Health Association's Herpes Resource Center and current managing editor of Sexual Health Communications.

Write to: American Social Health Association; Department T; P.O. Box 13827; Research Triangle Park, NC 27709; or phone (800) 230-6039.

Genital Herpes: A Patient Guide to Treatment
American Medical Association

No charge

This 32-page booklet has been prepared by the American Medical Association in consultation with leading STD clinicians and researchers, including the authors of *Herpes Controlled.* It offers a good overview of basic information on all aspects of genital herpes — an excellent quick reference. Your doctor or a local STD clinic may have copies on hand for distribution; if not, contact the AMA at one of the addresses listed below.

Write to: R. Mark Evans, PhD; American Medical Association; Healthcare Education Products; 515 North State Street; Chicago, IL 60610; or e-mail mark_evans@ama-assn.org.

Understanding Herpes
American Social Health Association

$6.00

This 20-page pamphlet focuses on the questions and concerns of newly diagnosed patients. An order includes two other ASHA publications, "Telling Your Partner" and "When Your Partner Has Herpes," and an index of back issues of *the helper.*

The Truth About Herpes, 4th edition
Stephen L. Sacks, MD

$24.95

A perennial favorite, now in its fourth edition, this book is a comprehensive guide to genital herpes, written in a straightforward, easy-to-read style. Abridged sections of this book are available as online patient handouts, free of charge, at the Viridae website. Dr. Sacks is a Canadian physician specializing in sexually transmitted diseases. Viridae is a contract research organization specializing in the development of antiviral drugs and vaccines.

Write to: Verdant Press; 1134 Burrard Street; Vancouver, BC V6Z 1Y8; or visit the Viridae website at www.viridae.com/publicns to download a faxable order form.

the helper
American Social Health Association
$25/year

This quarterly newsletter focuses on providing emotional and psychological support for people with herpes. It is a good source of information about coping with the disease and includes up-to-date general information and news of developments in herpes research.

Write to: American Social Health Association; Department T; P.O. Box 13827; Research Triangle Park, NC 27709; or phone (800) 230-6039.

Living with Herpes: The Facts and the Feelings
American Social Health Association
$19.95

An 18-minute video explaining basic aspects of genital herpes and addressing what it means to live with the disease.

5.3 WORLDWIDE WEB

In preparing this section, we looked for the word "herpes" on the Web using the AltaVista search engine. Initially, we retrieved more than 42,000 entries. Of course, such an unqualified search would be expected to turn up every indexed document or website where the word appears, regardless of its relevance, but our results should give you an idea just how extensively the subject is represented.

There are roughly a dozen herpes-related websites that you might want to investigate initially. Some are better than others. Some are, at best, suspect. The open quality of the web is its greatest strength and its greatest weakness. Any group or individual with a PC, a modem, and an ax to grind can set up a website and represent themselves as experts. Caution is advised with regard to any medical advice or information you find in cyberspace. Be especially wary of apparent public service sites shilling for "snake oil."

The inclusion of a site in the list that follows should in no way be regarded as an endorsement or recommendation unless otherwise stated in the description.

Sexual Health Communications   www.advicecenter.com

Operated by Sexual Health Communications, this site offers excellent summaries of the latest information about genital herpes and, more importantly, provides listings of clinics around the country with special expertise in genital herpes and other sexual health issues. The site also lists clinical trials that are seeking recruits and provides a way to contact the institutions or clinics doing research.

American Social Health Association   www.ashastd.org

As a national nonprofit devoted exclusively to STDs, the American Social Health Association (ASHA) has a wide range of educational publications, including a series of brochures on genital herpes and a quarterly herpes newsletter. Visitors to the website can access text for the brochures and sample articles from the newsletter. They can also find a list of local support groups affiliated with ASHA along with other resources.

Viridae   www.viridae.com/publicns

Viridae's website is one of the best online sources of accurate, up-to-date general information on genital herpes. Viridae is a Canadian contract research organization that develops antiviral drugs and vaccines for the pharmaceutical industry. The online patient information materials available from this site are abridged from Dr. Stephen L. Sacks' book, *The Truth About Herpes.*

Features:
- General information on herpes — a full range of subjects
- Links to other virology information sources

Herpeshelp   www.herpeshelp.com

Posted by the pharmaceutical firm Glaxo Wellcome, the manufacturer of acyclovir and valacyclovir, this site offer links to basic information on genital herpes and other STDs. It also gives detailed information about antiviral therapy and offers a discount coupon for Valtrex.®

Herpes: The Hidden Disease
www.azstarnet.com/~joanna/Herpes

A good source of general information with many links to other resources, this site was started and is maintained by a medical writer and motorcycle enthusiast in Arizona named Joanna Strohn. She undertook the project initially as a favor to a friend with herpes who was having difficulty finding information on the disease.

Features:
- Links to other sites providing information on diagnosis and treatment
- Link to information on the Herpes Resource Center and regional HELP groups
- Questions and answers about genital herpes from Columbia University's information service, "Go Ask Alice"
- Information of special interest to women
- E-mail subscription list for the anonymous exchange of questions and information in a public forum
- Links to support/social groups for people with genital herpes
- A bulletin board for comments, suggestions, questions, etc.

Arnot Ogden Medical Center www.aomc.org/herpes

This site is part of the Arnot Ogden Medical Center's "Health on Demand" catalog.

Features:
- Search engine
- Links to other sites providing information on genital herpes
- Information of special interest to women
- What women should know about sexually transmitted diseases (STDs), with information on chlamydia, herpes, gonorrhea, papillomavirus/genital warts, and syphilis. Includes links to other STD sites.

Café Herpé www.cafeherpe.com

This commercial site belongs to SmithKline Beecham, the manufacturers of famciclovir.

Features:
- Search engine
- General information on genital herpes
- General information on virology
- Information about famciclovir
- Links to related sites and herpes-oriented newsgroups

International Herpes Management Forum
www.pps.co.uk/ihmf/welcome

A good source of information on genital herpes. The IHMF is an international organization steered by some of the world's leading names in herpes research and dedicated to improving the standard of care for people with herpesvirus infections.

The Herpes Homepage   **www.minn.net/racoon/herpes**

Features:
- General information on herpes and links to other sites
- Information on conventional and alternative therapies
- Information about ongoing research
- Chat room
- Open Forum—a bulletin board to anonymously post and answer questions and exchange information with other people with herpes
- Link to dating service for people with herpes
- Support for partners of people with herpes
- Link to **alt.herpes.personals** newsgroup

Herpes: The Evasive Intruder
www.inet-access.net/~herpes

Features:
- Chat room
- General information on genital herpes
- Information on conventional and alternative therapies

Herpes Zone www.worldpassage.net/herpeszone

Features:

- General information on herpes
- Links to other sites

National Institute of Allergy and Infectious Diseases
www.nau.edu/~fronske/herpes

General information on genital herpes and other herpesvirus infections; no links.

Project Inform: Herpes Hotline Handout
www.projinfo.org/hh/herpes

Project Inform is a private nonprofit effort that focuses on HIV; includes information on genital herpes in the greater context of HIV infection and AIDS.

University of Illinois at Urbana-Champaign,
McKinley Health Center
www.uiuc.edu/departments/mckinley/health-info/
discond/commdis/genherpe

Questions and answers about genital herpes; no links.

Herpes Self-Help Group (America Online)

The AOL chat on herpes meets Tuesdays at 10:00 p.m. EST. Part of AOL's Better Health and Medical Network. Keyword: Better health

5.4 Organizations

American Social Health Association (ASHA)
P.O. Box 13827
Research Triangle Park, NC 27709

ASHA is a private nonprofit organization dedicated to the prevention and management of sexually transmitted diseases. Among its many services, ASHA coordinates the establishment of local support groups (HELP groups) in many cities around the country. To learn if there is a HELP group in your area, or to find out about establishing a local chapter, contact ASHA at the address listed above. ASHA also operates several herpes-related hotlines and is an excellent source of printed materials on genital herpes (see above).

appendix a

NONGENITAL
HSV INFECTIONS

≈

A.1 HSV INFECTIONS OF THE MOUTH AND THROAT

Acute herpetic gingivostomatitis (an infection of the mouth and gums) is the most common form of primary HSV-1 infection in children but is increasingly common among young adults. It is usually seen in young children, six months to five years of age. It produces painful reddening and swelling of the gums, which become delicate and bleed easily. Shallow ulcers appear mainly on the mucous lining of the mouth, on and under the tongue, and on the inner surfaces of the lips. Fever, drooling, heavy salivation, swollen glands, and extremely bad breath are common. Large quantities of virus are present in the saliva, and care should be taken to avoid accidental transmission of the infection from the mouth to the eyes. The disease is self-limiting (goes away on its own), but it may take several weeks for all symptoms to disappear. Symptoms in adults are similar to those seen in children, although they tend to be less severe. Pharyngitis (sore throat) is almost always seen in adults but is less common in children. Recurrent infection usually takes the form of cold sores or fever blisters.

Acute herpetic pharyngotonsillitis is the most common form of primary HSV-1 infection in adults, although HSV-2 can also cause this type of tonsillitis. Symptoms at onset include fever, malaise (a vague feeling of bodily discomfort), headache, and sore throat. Ulcers may appear on the tonsils. A yellowish-gray exudate will appear on the tonsils and in the back of the throat in about 50 percent of cases. In appearance, HSV pharyngotonsillitis is identical to strep throat; it is also easily confused with mononucleosis. Recurrent infection usually takes the form of cold sores or fever blisters.

Herpes labialis (cold sores or fever blisters on the mouth) is the principal manifestation of recurrent HSV infection of the mouth and throat. Most patients experience a **prodrome** (preliminary symptoms) of pain — burning, itching, tingling, or numbness at the site where the cold sore eventually appears. The prodromal phase usually precedes the appearance of lesions by about 6 hours but may last 24–48 hours. The most common site at which lesions appear is the lip (95 percent). Other sites include the nose, chin, and cheek. The lesions typically begin as a small cluster of reddened bumps that rapidly become fluid-filled vesicles. The vesicles become blister-like **pustules** and then crust over in a couple of days. Healing is usually complete within 6–10 days. Most people have less than two recurrences per year. Lesions usually appear in the same location each time and may be triggered by fever, stress, menstruation, and exposure to strong sunlight.

A.2 HSV Ocular (Eye) Infection

The most important common medical consequence of oral HSV-1 infection is probably ocular herpes — infection of the cornea and other tissues of the eye. This occurs in about 5 percent of people who have oral HSV-1 infections. The trigeminal ganglia of the face are divided into three sections, one of which innervates the region of the eye. If HSV-1 establishes latency in this section of the trigeminal ganglia, it can reactivate and cause recurrent ulceration of the cornea, known as corneal herpes or herpetic keratitis.

Primary HSV ocular infection is usually confined to one eye. Signs and symptoms include inflammation and swelling of the eyelid and the conjunctiva (the membrane lining the eyelid and surrounding the eyeball). Vesicles may form on the edges of the eyelid and other skin around the eye. Excessive watering of the eyes is common, and the patient may show an aversion to strong light. Most cases clear up on their own in two to three weeks. More than 25 percent of people with symptomatic primary HSV infection of the eye experience recurrent episodes. When ocular HSV infection recurs, it is usually in the form of inflammation of the cornea, eyelid, or conjunctiva. Repeated recurrences may lead to scarring of the cornea, the proliferation of new blood vessels in the eye, and eventual blindness.

Ocular HSV infection can also be acquired during childbirth when a newborn is exposed to HSV (usually HSV-2) in the mother's genital secretions.

A.3 HSV DERMATOLOGIC (SKIN) INFECTIONS

Ordinary epidermis, like the skin on your face or forearm, is protected from HSV infection by a very thin outer layer of hardened cells called the **stratum corneum.** Except on the soles of the feet and palms of the hands, this layer is only a few cells thick and is easily breached by minor cuts and scrapes or by a skin disease or exfoliative skin condition like eczema. Any break in the stratum corneum offers a potential portal of entry for HSV.

Traumatic herpes includes primary HSV skin infections that are not the result of autoinoculation during a primary oral or genital infection, but instead are caused when injured skin comes in contact with infectious virus. Athletes whose sports produce scrapes and abrasions and involve periods of prolonged direct physical contact are at risk. In wrestlers, true primary HSV skin infection is called herpes gladiatorum; in rugby players, it's known as scrumpox.

Herpetic whitlow is an extremely painful infection of the fingertip. In children, it's usually caused by thumb- or finger-sucking during a primary episode of oral HSV-1 infection. Similarly, in adults, some cases result from fingernail-biting, while others are caused by HSV-2 and result from touching the genitals during a primary episode of genital herpes. Recurrent whitlow tends to be just as painful as the primary infection but is usually of shorter duration. Historically, dental and medical professionals have been at high risk for herpetic whitlow because their hands are in frequent contact with contaminated saliva and secretions from patients with herpes. Today, however, as a result of the AIDS epidemic, latex gloves are worn during most procedures, reducing the risk of infection considerably. Herpetic whitlow can occur in a person with HSV antibodies, but as in most cases of HSV autoinoculation, it is far more likely to occur in conjunction with a primary oral or genital infection.

A.4 HSV Infection of the Central Nervous System

Herpes simplex encephalitis is an extremely rare but deadly inflammation of the brain. There are only about 1,000 cases each year in the United States, but without antiviral therapy, 70 percent of those who are infected will die. Roughly 50 percent are true primary infections, and 50 percent occur as a complication of recurrent infection, but the course and severity are the same in either case.

Herpes simplex meningitis is a relatively rare inflammation of the meninges (the membranes that cover the brain and spinal cord). It is usually benign and seen in adults as a complication of primary genital infection with HSV-2. In children, it is usually caused by HSV-1. Over 30 percent of women and about 10 percent of men with primary genital herpes develop meningitis. Symptoms include fever, stiff neck, severe headache, and aversion to bright light. Most cases are benign and brief, but associated symptoms of muscle weakness, difficult urination, numbness, and tingling may linger for several months. Aseptic meningitis (no HSV detectable in the spinal fluid) recurs in 20 to 30 percent of patients, most often accompanying a recurrence of genital herpes. Recurrent episodes tend to be milder symptomatically than the first episode.

A.5 Disseminated HSV Infection and HSV Infection in the Immunocompromised

The term **viremia** refers to the presence of virus in the bloodstream. Some degree of viremia is probably present during all primary HSV infections, but the body's natural defenses prevent the spread of infection to other anatomic sites. Very rarely, however, HSV in the bloodstream causes a more widespread or **disseminated** infection that can affect the entire skin or several internal organs. A disseminated HSV infection of the skin resembles an attack of measles. It is usually harmless and self-limiting and disappears in one to two weeks. Disseminated HSV infection of the internal organs, on the other hand, though rare, can be fatal. Several organs may be involved, but the liver is usually the most severely affected. Disseminated HSV infection is an *extremely rare* but often fatal condition in pregnancy, usually occurring in the third trimester. The death rate for mother and fetus exceeds 50 percent. Immunocompromised patients are the most susceptible to disseminated infection.

A person's immune system can be suppressed or compromised by a number of conditions and circumstances. Immunocompromise can be an inborn trait, or it can induced by disease (cancer, AIDS), injury (burns), malnutrition, or immunosuppressive drugs given to transplant recipients. Immunocompromised patients are at increased risk for severe and sometimes fatal HSV infection—both primary and recurrent.

A.6 Neonatal Herpes
(HSV Infection in the Newborn)

Neonatal HSV infection and its prevention are discussed in Section 2.7.

appendix b

Type-Specific Serologic Tests

$\sim$

Accurate tests that identify antibodies to HSV-1 and HSV-2 are useful in a variety of situations described in this book. For example, they may be utilized when sampling conditions are not adequate for a culture or antigen tests, or for diagnosing asymptomatic or "subclinical" infections, or to supplement other testing methods in cases where a patient has unusual symptoms.

Unfortunately for the health care consumer, getting an accurate test is not always easy. A number of commercial tests which claim to differentiate antibodies to HSV-1 from those to HSV-2 actually react with either type. Thus, the results are frequently inaccurate.

The HSV Western blot got around this problem by using HSV-1 and HSV-2 proteins which have been separated by size, so that type-specific antibody profiles can be recognized with a specificity of >99 percent. As such, it is the current gold standard in HSV serology.

Though it began exclusively as a research tool, the Western blot has been made available on a semi-commercial basis through the University of Washington Virology Laboratory. Readers of this book can obtain a Western blot by following the steps outlined below. In addition, a new type-specific serum test has recently received approval for marketing in the United States. You and your medical professional may find this more convenient for your needs. This test, called the POCkit HSV-2 Rapid Test, uses a fingerprick and blotter to identify HSV-2, with results available immediately in the health care provider's office. For information about how your medical professional can obtain the POCkit HSV-2 Rapid Test,™ you can call (877-7POCKIT) or visit the POCkit™ web site at www.diagnology.com. Additional diagnostic information is available from the Sexual Health Communications hotline (888-ADVICE8).

FIRST STEPS

To get a Western blot for yourself or a partner, you will first need to enlist the cooperation of your health care provider. For patient referrals to clinics that offer this test, patients can call Sexual Health Communications at 888-ADVICE8. Providers who aren't familiar with the test can contact the University of Washington Virology Laboratory for the most up-to-date instructions on how to draw a sample and ship it. The phone number—FOR HEALTH CARE PROFESSIONALS ONLY—is 206-526-2088.

The blood sample required for the test will be shipped in a leak-proof, unbreakable tube, shipped with ice packs by overnight courier or on dry ice.

TIME TO SEROCONVERSION

Paired sera run by Western blot will show seroconversion in 90 percent of HSV-1 patients and in 100 percent of HSV-2 patients by three months after infection. Antibodies can sometimes be detected earlier, however, and about 50 percent of people will "seroconvert" in two to three weeks. The median time to seroconversion for either Western blot or POCkit™ is 13 days.

TURNAROUND TIMES

Western blot results are available in 5–7 days from the time the serum arrives in the lab. A small number of samples require extra Western blot testing and will require 7–10 days.

For information and referrals, patients may call 888-ADVICE8.
Health care professionals may contact:

> University of Washington Virology Laboratory
> University of Washington Medical Center
> Room NW 220
> 1959 N.E. Pacific St., Seattle, WA 98195
> Phone: 206-526-2088
> Fax: 206-528-2793

References

Ashley, RL et al. Comparison of Western blot (immunoblot) and glycoprotein G-specific immunodot enzyme assay for detecting antibodies to herpes simplex virus types 1 and 2 in human sera. J Clin Micro; 26:662-667 (1988)

BIBLIOGRAPHY

~

Alford CA, Britt WJ. Cytomegalovirus. In: Roizman B, Whitley RJ, Lopez C, eds. *The Human Herpesviruses.* New York, NY: Raven Press;1993: 227–255.

Benedetti J, Corey L, Ashley R. Recurrence rates in genital herpes after symptomatic first-episode infection. *Ann Intern Med.* 1994;121:847–854.

Brown Z, Selke S, Zeh J, et al. The acquisition of herpes simplex virus during pregnancy. *New Engl J Med.* 1997;337:509–515.

Bryson Y, Dillon M, Bernstein DI, Radolf J, Zakowski P, Garratty E. Risk of acquisition of genital herpes simplex virus type 2 in sex partners of persons with genital herpes: a prospective couple study. *J Infect Dis.* 1993;167;942–946.

Catotti DN, Clarke P, Catoe KE. Herpes revisited: still a cause for concern. *Sexually Trans Dis.* 1993;20:77–80.

Centers for Disease Control. Diseases characterized by genital ulcers. *MMWR Morb Mortal Wkly Rep.* 1998;47:18–26.

Corey L. Genital Herpes. In: Holmes KH, Mårdh P-A, Sparling PF, Wiesner PJ, eds. *Sexually Transmitted Diseases.* 2nd ed. New York, NY: McGraw-Hill, Inc;1990:391–413.

De Lellis L, Fabris M, Cassai E, et al. Herpesvirus-like DNA sequences in non-AIDS Kaposi's sarcoma. *J Infect Dis.* 1995;172:1605–1607.

Drugs for non-HIV viral infection. *Med Lett.* 1994;36:27–30.

Famvir® (famciclovir) full prescribing information.

Fleming DT, McQuillan GM, Johnson RF, et al. Herpes simplex virus type 2 in the United States, 1976 to 1994. *New Engl J Med.* 1997;337:1105–1111.

Gentry GA, Lowe M, Alford G, Nevins R. Sequence analyses of herpesviral enzymes suggest an ancient origin for human sexual behavior. *Proc Natl Acad Sci USA.* 1988;85:2658–2661.

Goldberg LH, Kaufman R, Kurtz TO, et al. Long-term suppression of recurrent genital herpes with acyclovir. *Arch Dermatol.* 1993;129:582–587.

Herpes: the new sexual leprosy. *Time.* July 28, 1980:76.

Karcher DS, Alkan S. Herpes-like DNA sequences, AIDS-related tumors, and cattleman's disease. *New Engl J Med.* 1995;333:797–798. Letter.

Langenberg, AGM, Burke RL, Adair S, Sekulovich R, Dekker C, Corey L. A recombinant glycoprotein vaccine for herpes simplex type 2: Safety and immunogenicity. *Ann Intern Med.* 1995;122:889–898.

Leo J. The new scarlet letter. *Time.* August 2,1982:62–66.

Liebowitz D, Kieff E. Epstein-Barr virus. In: Roizman B, Whitley RJ, Lopez C, eds. *The Human Herpesviruses.* New York, NY: Raven Press; 1993:107–172.

Mertz GJ, Jones CC, Mills J, et al. Long-term acyclovir suppression of frequently recurring genital herpes simplex virus infection. *JAMA.* 1988;260:201–206.

Oxman MN. Genital herpes. In: Gorbach SL, Bartlett JG, Blacklow NR, eds. *Infectious Diseases.* Philadelphia, PA: W. B. Saunders Company; 1992:828–845.

Oxman MN. Herpes simplex viruses and human herpesvirus 6. In: Gorbach SL, Bartlett JG, Blacklow NR, eds. *Infectious Diseases.* Philadelphia, PA: W. B. Saunders Company;1992:1667–1700.

Roizman B. The family herpesviridae: a brief introduction. In: Roizman B, Whitley RJ, Lopez C, eds. *The Human Herpesviruses.* New York, NY: Raven Press;1993:1–9.

Valtrex® (valacyclovir hydrochloride) full prescribing information.

Wald A, Zeh J, Barnum G, Davis LG, Corey L. Suppression of subclinical shedding of herpes simplex virus type 2 with acyclovir. *Ann Intern Med.* 1996;124:8–15.

Whitley RJ, Gnann JW. The epidemiology and clinical manifestations of herpes simplex virus infections. In: Roizman B, Whitley RJ, Lopez C, eds. *The Human Herpesviruses.* New York, NY: Raven Press; 1993:69–105.

Zovirax® (acyclovir) full prescribing information.

INDEX

~

Note: Page numbers followed by *f* indicate illustrations; page numbers followed by *t* indicate tables.

Acyclovir
  costs of, 128–129
  effectiveness of, 89, 126
  generic versions of, 89, 128–129
  in primary infections, 89–90, 90t
  in recurrent infections
    in episodic therapy, 94, 94t, 127
    in suppressive therapy, 95–96, 95t,
      97t, 106, 127
  safety profile of, 90–91, 128
  in transmission prevention, 98
Adenopathy. *See* Swollen glands
Adverse events, with drugs, 90–91,
  127–128
Age, as risk factor, 53, 56t
AIDS
  genital herpes with, 54
  testing for, 69
Alternative medicine, 106–110
Anal sex, virus transmission in, 27
  proctitis in, 71t
Animals, herpesviruses of, 21, 24
Antibodies, viral, 32
  appearance of (seroconversion), 154–155

serologic tests for, 68–69, 153–155
Antigens, viral
  detection of, 67
  immune response to, 31–35, 131
Antiviral drugs. *See also* Acyclovir;
    Famciclovir; Valacyclovir
  adverse events with, 90–91, 127–128
  clinical trials of, 107–108
  costs of, 128–129
  effectiveness of, 87–88, 126
  in primary infections, 88–91, 90t
  recurrence rate and, 64
  in recurrent infections
    episodic, 93–94, 94t, 98–100,
      126–127
    suppressive, 93, 95–100, 95t, 97t, 106,
      127
  safety profile of, 90–91, 127–128
  in transmission prevention, 98, 104
Appetite loss, in genital herpes, 58, 122
Asymptomatic infections, 36, 48, 52,
    122
  epidemiology of, 55, 61
  in partner, 130–131
  viral transmission during, 52
Asymptomatic viral shedding. *See* Viral
    shedding
Athletes, herpetic skin infections in, 149

Autoinoculation, 28, 30, 123
  herpetic whitlow in, 27

Barrier protection
  with cold sores, 132–133
  in genital herpes prevention, 100–104,
    130
Behavioral characteristics, genital herpes
    risk in, 53–55, 56t
Blisters. See Vesicles
Blood tests. See Serologic tests
Brain, herpes simplex infections of, 60t,
    150
Burning, in genital herpes, 57, 63

Capsids, of herpesviruses, 21f
Capsomeres, of herpesviruses, 21f
Central nervous system, herpetic infec-
    tions of, 60t, 150
Cervical lesions, 57, 60t
  necrosis of, 70t
  viral replication in, 58
Childbirth, in active genital herpes,
    delivery methods for, 73, 105–106
Children
  herpetic gingivostomatitis in, 147
  herpetic whitlow in, 149
  viral transmission in, 26
Chlamydia infections, testing for, 69
Clinical trials, of genital herpes treat-
    ments, 107–108
Cocaine use, genital herpes risk and, 56t
Cold sores
  genital HSV-1 infection immunity in,
    33, 131–132
  healing of, 148
  oral sex and, 130
  prodrome of, 132
  serotypes causing, 36
  viral transmission in, 132–133
Communication, about genital herpes
    status, 3, 102–103, 133
Complications, of genital herpes, non-
    genital, 69, 70t–71t, 147–151
Condoms, in genital herpes prevention,
    100–104, 129, 130
Conjunctivitis, in ocular infections, 148

Corneal herpetic infections, 148–149
Counseling, 86
Crusts, on lesions, 29f, 57, 63t
Culture, viral, 66–67
Cunnilingus
  barrier protection in, 100, 103–104
  virus transmission in, 27–28
Cytomegalovirus infections, 23t

Demographics, of genital herpes, 53–55,
    56t
Depression, in genital herpes, 85–86, 87f
Dermatologic infections. See Skin
"Dew drops on a rose petal" lesions, 61,
    122
Diagnosis, 65–69
  antigen-detection tests in, 67
  of concurrent sexually transmitted dis-
    eases, 69
  direct fluorescence antibody testing in, 67
  emotional impact of, 85–87, 87f
  history in, 65
  in partner, 131
  physical examination in, 66
  polymerase chain reaction in, 68, 125
  serologic testing in, 68–69, 153–155
  Tzanck test in, 68
  viral culture in, 66–67
Diary, herpes, 92, 124
Dietary treatment, of recurrent infec-
    tions, 109–110
Direct fluorescence antibody testing, 67
Discordant couples, viral transmission
    in, 52–53
Disseminated herpetic infections,
    150–151
Dormant state, 30
  reactivation from, 30–31, 124
  triggering factors in, 30, 92, 124–125
Double-blind trials, of antiviral drugs, 107
Drooling, in herpetic gingivostomatitis,
    147

Education, genital herpes risk and, 56t
Educational materials. See Resources
Emotional impact, of genital herpes, 2–3,
    70t, 85–87

Encephalitis, herpes simplex, 150
Envelope, of herpesviruses, 21f
Enzyme immunoassay, for herpes simplex virus, 154–155
Epidemiology
of genital herpes, 49–51, 51t
asymptomatic, 55
risk factors and, 53–55, 56t
of neonatal herpes, 71–72
Epidermis, resistance of, to viral penetration, 25–26, 149
Episodic therapy, for genital herpes, 93–94, 94t, 98–100, 126–127
Epstein-Barr virus, 22, 23t
Ethnic groups, genital herpes epidemiology in, 51, 51t, 55
Exogenous reinfection, 131
Eye, herpetic infections of, 148–149

Famciclovir
absorption of, 89
advantages of, 90
costs of, 128–129
effectiveness of, 126
in primary infections, 89–90, 90t, 110
in recurrent infections, 94t, 95t
safety profile of, 90–91, 128
Famvir.® See Famciclovir
Fear, in genital herpes, 85–86, 87f
Feelings, about genital herpes, 2–3, 70t, 85–87
Fellatio
barrier protection in, 100, 103–105
virus transmission in, 27–28
Fever
in genital herpes, 58, 60t, 61t, 122
in herpetic gingivostomatitis, 147
viral reactivation in, 30, 92
Fever blisters. See Cold sores
Fingertip, herpetic whitlow of, 149–150
recurrent, 149
viral transmission in, 27, 28

Ganglia, virus latency in, 30, 31f, 32f
Gay women, viral transmission in, 132–133
Gender. See also Men; Women

as risk factor, 53–54
Gingivostomatitis, herpetic, 147
Glycoprotein spikes, of herpesviruses, 21f, 154
Gonorrhea
genital herpes transmission in, 54
testing for, 69
Gums, herpetic infections of, 147

Headache, in genital herpes, 58, 60t, 61t, 122
Healing
of cold sores, 148
of genital lesions, 60t, 63t, 125
Herpes gladiatorum, 149
Herpes labialis. See Cold sores
Herpes simplex virus type 1 (HSV-1)
antigens of, immune response to, 32–35
diseases associated with, 22, 23t
evolution of, 24
in genital infections, 24, 26–27
epidemiology of, 50
immunity to, 33
recurrent patterns in, 64, 91
transmission of, 129–130
herpes simplex virus type 2 compared with
antigens, 32–35
sites affected, 24–25, 132
partial immunity to, 48
transmission of, 26–27, 123
Herpes simplex virus type 2 (HSV-2)
antigens of, immune response to, 32–35
diseases associated with, 22, 23t
evolution of, 24
herpes simplex virus type 1 compared with
antigens, 32–35
sites affected, 24–25, 132
in oral infections, transmission of, 129–130
partial immunity to, 33–35, 48
survival on environmental surfaces, 26
transmission of, 27–28
Herpesvirus family, 21–22, 21f
human, 22, 23t

Herpetic whitlow, 149–150
  recurrent, 149
  viral transmission in, 27, 28
Historical review, of genital herpes,
    47–49
History, medical, 65
Holistic remedies, 106–110
Hotlines, 137–138
HSV. See Herpes simplex virus
Human herpesvirus 6 infections, 23t
Human herpesvirus 7 infections, 23t
Human herpesvirus 8 infections, 23t
Human herpesvirus family, 22, 23t
Human immunodeficiency virus infection
  genital herpes with, 54
  testing for, 69

Immune response, to viral antigens,
    31–35, 123, 131
  partial immunity in, 33–35, 48,
    131–132
Immunocompromise, herpetic infections
    in, 22
  disseminated, 150–151
  exogenous reinfections in, 131
Incidence, of genital herpes, 49–51, 51t
Incurability, of genital herpes, 87–88,
    124
Infants, newborn. See Neonatal herpes
    infections
Information resources. See Resources
Injury
  herpetic skin infections in, 149
  viral reactivation in, 30, 92, 125
Inoculation, of virus, 28
  self-, 27, 28, 30, 123
Intercourse
  first age of, as risk factor, 53, 56t
  safer sex practices in. See Safer sex
    practices
  viral reactivation in, 92
  viral transmission in, 129–130
Itching, in genital herpes, 57, 59, 63, 63t

Kaposi's sarcoma, human herpesvirus 8
    in, 23t
Keratitis, herpetic, 148–149

Kissing, virus transmission in, 26,
    132–133

Latency, of viruses, 20, 22, 30, 124
  in sacral ganglia, 30, 31f
  serotypes and, 33
  in trigeminal ganglia, 30, 32f, 148–149
  vaccine development and, 110–111
Legal aspects, of genital herpes disclosure,
    102
Lesbians, viral transmission in, 132–133
Lesions. See also Vesicles
  distribution of
    in men, 59, 59f, 62, 63t
    in nonprimary infections, 60–61, 61t
    in primary infections, 57, 58f, 59, 59f,
      61t
    in recurrent infections, 61–62, 63t,
      125
    in women, 57, 58f, 62, 63t
  formation of, 28, 29f, 30, 57, 59
  surface area of, 60t, 63t
Lips, herpes infections of. See Cold sores
Lymph nodes, swelling of. See Swollen
    glands
Lysine, in recurrent infections, 109–110

Malaise, in genital herpes, 58, 60t, 61t,
    122
Malnutrition, viral reactivation in, 30
Marital status, genital herpes risk and,
    56t
Men, genital herpes in
  epidemiology of, 51, 51t
  primary, 59–60, 59f, 60t
  recurrent, 62, 63t
  symptoms of, 59–60, 59f, 60t, 62, 63t,
    122
  virus transmission to, 52–53
Meningitis, herpes simplex, 60t, 150
Menstruation, viral reactivation in, 30,
    92
Mouth, herpetic infections of, 147–148.
    See also Cold sores
Mucous membrane
  ulcers on, 28
  virus transmission through, 25

Muscle aches, in genital herpes, 58, 60t, 61t, 122
Myths, about genital herpes, 1–2

Natural remedies, 106–110
Necrotic cervicitis, 70t
Neonatal herpes infections, 71–73
  acquisition of, 72
  incidence of, 71–72
  management of, 72–73
  ocular, 149
  prevention of, 105–106
Nerve cells, herpes simplex virus in, 22
Nongenital herpes infections, 147–151
  brain, 60t, 150
  disseminated, 150–151
  eye, 148–149
  in immunocompromise, 150–151
  mouth, 147–148. *See also* Cold sores
  in recurrent genital herpes, 63t
  skin, 149–150. *See also* Herpetic whitlow
Nonprimary infections, 35, 48, 60–61, 61t

Ocular herpetic infections, 148–149
On-line information sources, 140–144
Oral sex
  barrier protection in, 100, 103–105
  with cold sores, 130, 132–133
  viral transmission in, 27–28, 50, 129–130, 132–133
Organizations, for support groups, 144–145
Outbreaks. *See* Recurrent infections

Pain
  in anorectal herpes, 71t
  in genital herpes
    in men, 59, 60t, 61t, 62, 63t
    prodromal, 63
    recurrent, 63, 63t
    in women, 57–58, 60t, 61t, 62, 63t
  in herpetic gingivostomatitis, 147
  in herpetic whitlow, 149
Papules, appearance of, 29f
Partial immunity, to other serotype, 33–35, 48, 131–132
Pathogenesis, of infections, 28, 29f, 30

Patterns of recurrence, in genital herpes, 64, 91–92, 124
Penciclovir, 89
Penis, lesions on, 59–60, 59f, 62
Pharyngitis, herpetic, 71t, 147–148
Physical examination, 66
POCkit HSV-2 Rapid Test, 69, 154
Polymerase chain reaction, in viral detection, 68, 125
Pregnancy, herpetic infections in
  disseminated, 151
  transmission to fetus and newborn, 71–73, 105–106
  viral shedding in, 105–106
Prevalence, of genital herpes, 49–51, 51t
Prevention
  of cold sores, barrier methods in, 132–133
  of genital herpes, 100–106
    antiviral drugs in, 98, 104
    barrier methods in, 100–104, 130
    in monogamous relationship, with one herpes-positive partner, 103–105
    in oral sex, 129–130
    in pregnancy, 105–106
    in single, sexually active, nonmonogamous relationship
      with genital herpes, 102–103
      with no genital herpes history, 100–102
    suppressive therapy in, 93, 95–100, 95t, 97t, 106, 127, 129
Primary infections
  complications of, 69, 70t–71t
  definition of, 35, 48
  historical review of, 48
  recurrent infections presenting as, 123
  symptoms of, 57–60, 58f, 59f, 60t, 61t, 122
  treatment of, 88–91, 90t
  viral spread during, 28, 29f, 30
Proctitis, 71t
Prodrome
  of cold sores, 132, 148
  of genital herpes, 62–64
    episodic therapy in, 126–127
    recognition of, 91–92, 93, 124

Prophylactic (suppressive) therapy, for genital herpes, 93, 95–100, 95t, 97t, 106, 127, 129
Psychosocial aspects, of genital herpes, 2–3, 70t, 85–87
Publications, 138–140
Pustules
appearance of, 29f
in cold sores, 148

Race, genital herpes epidemiology and, 51, 51t, 55
Reactivation, of virus, 30–31, 124
triggering factors in, 30, 92, 124–125
Recurrent infections (genital), 91–100. See also Reactivation, of viruses
patterns of, 64, 91–92, 124
prediction of, 93
in pregnancy, 73
presenting as primary infection, 123
prodrome recognition in, 91–92, 93
symptoms of, 61–62, 63t, 121, 125
prevention and reduction of, 95–96, 97t
treatment of, 91–100
asymptomatic viral shedding reduction in, 96, 98
diary in, 92, 124
episodic therapy in, 93–94, 94t, 98–100, 126–127
prodrome recognition in, 91–92, 93
suppressive therapy in, 93, 95–100, 95t, 97t, 106, 127, 129
symptomatic recurrence reduction in, 95–96, 97t
viral shedding in, 62, 96, 98
Recurrent infections (nongenital or unspecified)
herpetic whitlow, 149
likelihood of, 25, 91
meningitis, 150
ocular, 148
after reactivation, 31
Redness, of skin, 28
Reinfection, exogenous, 131
Replication, of viruses
after inoculation, 28

in nerve cells, 30
time pattern of, 58
Resources, 137–145
hotlines, 137–138
organizations, 144–145
publications, 138–140
videos, 140
websites, 140–144
Risk factors, for viral transmission, 53–55, 56t
to neonates, 72
Rural vs. urban population, genital herpes risk and, 56t

Sacral ganglia, viral latency in, 30, 31f, 110
Safer sex practices, 130–131
with cold sores, 132–133
in discordant couple, 103–105
with genital herpes diagnosis, 102–103
with no genital herpes history, 100–101
in pregnancy, 106
Saliva, virus transmission in, 26–27, 147
Semen, virus transmission in, 27
Seroconversion, time to, 154–155
Serologic tests, 68–69, 153–155
accuracy of, 153–154
how to obtain, 154
rapid, 69, 154
seroconversion time and, 154–155
turnaround times for, 155
Serotypes, of viruses, 33
Sexual activity. See also Intercourse; Oral sex; Safer sex practices
avoidance of, during symptomatic episode, 102, 103
number of years of, as risk factor, 55
Sexual partners
asymptomatic infections in, 130–131
herpes infection identification in, 130–131
number of, as risk factor, 53, 56t, 101
telling about genital herpes status, 3, 102–103, 133
Sexually transmitted diseases
risk factors for, 53–55, 56t

testing for, 69
Shedding, viral. *See* Viral shedding
Side effects, of drugs, 90–91
Skin
  herpetic infections of, 149–150. *See also* Herpetic whitlow
  in disseminated disease, 150–151
  virus penetration of, 25–26, 28
Socioeconomic status, viral transmission and, 26, 54, 56t
Sore throat, herpetic, 71t, 147–148
Spermicides, genital herpes transmission and, 101
Spinal cord, herpetic meningitis of, 150
Sports, herpetic skin infections in, 149
Strains, of viruses, 33, 131
Stress, viral reactivation in, 30, 92, 125
Subclinical viral shedding. *See* Viral shedding
Sunburn, viral reactivation in, 30, 92, 125
Superinfections, in genital herpes, 70t
Support groups, 86, 144–145
Suppressive therapy, for genital herpes, 93, 95–100, 95t, 97t, 106, 127, 129
Swollen glands
  in genital herpes, in men, 58, 59, 60t, 62, 63t, 122
  in herpetic gingivostomatitis, 147
Symptomatic infections, definition of, 48
Symptoms, of genital herpes, 121–122
  appearance after sexual contact, 57
  constitutional
    in nonprimary infections, 60–61, 61t
    in primary infections, 58, 59, 60t, 61t, 122
  duration of
    in nonprimary infections, 61t
    in primary infections, 59–60, 60t
    in recurrent infections, 61–62, 63t, 125
  lack of. *See* Asymptomatic infections
  local, 58
  in men, 59–60, 59f, 60t, 62, 63t, 122
  mild, 48, 55, 121
  in nonprimary infections, 60–61, 61t
  in pregnancy, delivery method and, 73

  in primary infections, 57–60, 58f, 59f, 60t, 61t, 122
  prodromal, 62–64, 91–92, 93, 124
  in recurrent infections, 61–62, 63t, 121
    prevention and reduction of, 95–96, 97t
  severity of, 55, 61
  sexual activity during, 102, 103
  sudden appearance of, 123
  in type 1 infection, 57
  unrecognized, 48, 55, 122, 123
  in women, 57–58, 58f, 60t, 62, 63t, 122
Syphilis
  genital herpes transmission in, 54
  testing for, 69

Tegument, of herpesviruses, 21f
Telephone hotlines, 137–138
Tonsillitis, herpetic, 71t, 147–148
Transmission, of infections, 52–53, 123
  autoinoculation in, 27, 28, 30, 123
  in children, 26
  concerns about, 98
  in discordant couples, 52–53
  fear of, 86, 87f
  herpes simplex virus-1, 26–27
  herpes simplex virus-2, 27–28
  to newborn, 72–73, 149
  in oral sex, 27–28, 50, 129–130, 132–133
  prevention of. *See* Prevention, of genital herpes
  risk factors for, 53–55, 56t, 72
  routes for, 25–26
  spermicides and, 101
  in viral shedding, 102, 125
Trauma
  herpetic skin infections in, 149
  viral reactivation in, 30, 92, 125
Treatment, of genital herpes, 85–112. *See also* Antiviral drugs; *specific drugs*
  alternative medicine in, 106–110
  dietary, 109–110
  drug approval process and, 106–110
  patient control in, 92
  preventive, 100–106
  primary, 88–91, 90t
  recurrent, 91–100

in asymptomatic viral shedding reduction, 96, 98
diary in, 92, 124
episodic therapy in, 93–94, 94t,
98–100, 126–127
prodrome recognition in, 91–92, 93,
124
suppressive therapy in, 93, 95–100,
95t, 97t, 106, 127, 129
in symptomatic recurrence reduction,
95–96, 97t
research on, 110–112
Trigeminal ganglia, viral latency in, 30,
32f, 148–149
Triggering factors, in viral reactivation,
30, 92, 124–125
Tzanck test, 68

Ulcers
corneal, 148–149
formation of, 28, 29f
genital, appearance of, 57, 122
oral, 147
pharyngeal, 71t, 148
Unrecognized infections, 48, 55, 122, 123
Urban vs. rural population, genital herpes risk and, 56t
Urethral inflammation, in genital herpes,
57, 60t, 63t, 70t
Urination, painful, 57, 59, 60t, 63, 63t,
70t, 122

Vaccines, for genital herpes, 110–112
Vaginal discharge, in genital herpes, 27,
57, 60t, 63t
Valacyclovir
absorption of, 89
advantages of, 90
costs of, 128–129
effectiveness of, 126
in primary infections, 89–90, 90t
in recurrent infections, 94, 94t, 95t, 127
safety profile of, 90–91, 128
Valtrex.® See Valacyclovir
Varicella-zoster virus infections, 23t
Vesicles
appearance of, 29f
coalescence of, 57

in cold sores, 148
distribution and spreading of, in
women, 57, 58f, 63t
eyelid, 148
formation of, 28, 29f
virus autoinoculation from, 27, 28, 30
Videos, on herpes, 140
Viral culture, 66–67
Viral shedding, 124
from cold sores, 132
duration of, 125
frequency of, 126
in nonprimary infections, 60–61, 61t
in pregnancy, 105–106
in primary infections, 57, 59, 60t, 61t
in prodromal stage, 64
in reactivation, 30–31
in recurrent infections, 62, 63t, 96, 98
suppressive therapy for, 127
virus transmission during, 102
Viremia, 150
Virions, 20, 21, 21f
Viruses, general characteristics of, 19–20

Web sites, on genital herpes, 140–144
Western blot test, 68–69, 153–155
accuracy of, 153–154
how to obtain, 154
rapid, 69, 154
seroconversion time and, 154–155
turnaround times for, 155
Whitlow, herpetic, 149–150
recurrent, 149
viral transmission in, 27, 28
Women. See also Pregnancy
gay, viral transmission in, 132–133
genital herpes in
epidemiology of, 51, 51t
primary, 57–58, 58f, 60t
recurrent, 62, 63t
symptoms of, 57–58, 58f, 60t, 62, 63t,
122
vesicle distribution in, 57, 58f, 63t
virus transmission to, 52–54
Wrestlers, herpes gladiatorum in, 149

Zovirax.® See Acyclovir